Your Personal Best

A common sense guide to fitness for all ages

by

Marie McDonald

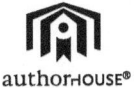

authorHOUSE®

AuthorHouse™
1663 Liberty Drive, Suite 200
Bloomington, IN 47403
www.authorhouse.com
Phone: 1-800-839-8640

First published by AuthorHouse 9/17/2007

ISBN: 978-1-4343-3370-4 (sc)

Library of Congress Control Number: 2007906151

Printed in the United States of America
Bloomington, Indiana

This book is printed on acid-free paper.

This book is dedicated to the YMCAs all over the world.
The "Y" inspired my passion for aquatics, which shaped my life.

Marie McDonald

ACKNOWLEDGEMENTS

My editor, Barbara Hudson, who not only helped me through this whole process, but patiently endured my lack of computer skills. I could not have done this without her.

Melanie Byrne and the Las Vegas Athletic Club for hiring a seventy-eight year old fitness professional – me.

My family and friends for their support and encouragement.

Terrisa Meeks and the Northwest Writers Group, where I expanded my writing skills.

CREDITS

Cover and swim team photo courtesy of Jim Atkins.

Back cover photo courtesy of Portraits Today by Catherine.

Snapshots at the Las Vegas Athletic Club taken by Terrisa Meeks and Helen Lam.

INTRODUCTION

Where would you look if you wanted to know the stages of development of the human body, both physically and mentally, from birth through old age? Include the changes that occur at each stage, and how to maintain a fitness level that could enable you to live a healthier, happier life.

If you need advice on weight control, you need to know the most sensible, effective method that actually works. Where would you find such advice? There are hundreds of diets and exercise programs out there today. The market is literally flooded with books, videos, gadgets and equipment designed to separate you from your money. The unfortunate result is usually disappointment. How do you decide what method to believe? The answer to that question is the source of the information. You must know there is sufficient proof that the source of the information is trustworthy.

Perhaps you have questions concerning fitness programs recommended for people with Arthritis or Osteoporosis. Are you aware there are even very successful programs for the severely handicapped and the disabled? The results are nothing short of miraculous! No, fitness programs cannot cure these conditions; however, in many cases they do improve the quality of life considerably, enabling increased ease and freedom of movement.

Maybe you are just interested in how best to maintain, or build, your fitness level during your journey through those "Golden Years." So many people convince themselves it is too late for change or improvement; however, it is not only possible, but rewarding and enjoyable as well.

Where would you find all this information? You could visit the nearest library and check out a stack of reference books – or you could simply open this book and start reading. One small book, written in simple, straightforward language that anyone can easily understand, could provide everything you require. Most of the subjects I have discussed here are one-subject books.

I could go on and on about all of the information in this book. Just peek at the contents page. You will get a glimpse of just how many subjects this one book encompasses. As the subtitle indicates, it is a *Common Sense Guide to Fitness for All Ages*.

The author, Marie McDonald, is not attempting to sell you anything. As she puts it, "I wrote the book because I have something to say. People ask me every day, how do you stay in such great shape? So, why not tell them."

Marie is a living, breathing testimonial to her own advice on achieving and maintaining a lifetime of fitness. Take a good look at the pictures of Marie – this is the real thing. The picture on the front cover is at age sixty-eight and the picture on the last page of the book is age seventy-nine. There have been no surgeries, or alterations. What you see is just an extremely fit, attractive lady who is also a mother, grandmother and great-grandmother! Amazing, isn't it?

Her accomplishments in the field of fitness are quite impressive. She has received numerous awards and recognition for her many achievements in the fitness field and, even though she has certainly earned the right to sit back and rest on her laurels, she continues to live the life of fitness she has practiced for more than seven decades.

There are a few of Marie's achievements and awards on the back cover of this book, however I would like to expand on that subject.

She is the proud owner of the *National ATT Silver Spirit Award* and earned eighty-nine medals and ribbons for Master and Senior State competitions. Gold, Silver and Bronze are the result of participating in the Senior Competitive Sports events, as well as setting pool records. The always-amazing Marie even won second runner up in the *Ms. Senior America Pageant.*

Her most recent award came as a complete surprise to Marie. A friend read about the contest and entered Marie without her knowledge. Marie remained completely unaware of the entry until the notification of the award as *Ageless Champion of 2007* for *Athletic Achievement*. Marie and three other winners, in other categories, accepted trophies at a recent awards luncheon. The complete coverage with photos will appear in the local publication, *The View,* the end of July. She is seventy-nine and still winning awards!

There are many other awards, recognitions and honors not listed here; I think you will agree Marie is an exceptional person. She is also a fully certified instructor in all the categories of fitness she teaches - plus numerous others over the years.

After a career of working with people from all walks of life, from children to the elderly; from the just out-of-shape, to the out-of-hope, the disabled and the handicapped, you might expect Marie McDonald to be sitting back enjoying those well-earned retirement years. That is what you might expect, but you would be wrong. Marie is still doing what she loves – helping people achieve fitness and better health. Three or four days a week you will find Marie doing 'business as usual', instructing her various groups at one of the largest and best equipped *Las Vegas Athletic Clubs* in the area. That's right - she is still working as a fitness instructor! As one photographer observed, "She never stops moving." Her energy and enthusiasm are truly amazing.

As I stated in the beginning, you need to have confidence and trust the source of your information. Who better to believe than someone that has spent her life living the advice she recommends for others? In other words, she practices what she preaches.

Barbara Hudson,
Las Vegas freelance writer and writing coach

**

Contents

INTRODUCTION   xi

PART ONE

SETTING GOALS   3
EXERCISE   6
   ABDOMINALS   10
   WEIGHT TRAINING   11
   WATER EXERCISE   13
   MIND/BODY   18
      AI CHI   19
      PILATES   22
      TAI CHI   23
      YOGA   24
SPORTS/DANCE   26
WEIGHT CONTROL/DIET   28
AGING   36
ARTHRITIS   41
OSTEOPOROSIS   47

PART TWO

BIRTH TO AGE SIX   55
SEVEN THROUGH TWELVE   62
THIRTEEN THROUGH EIGHTEEN   70
NINETEEN THROUGH FORTY   75
THE CHILDBEARING YEARS   82
FORTY-ONE THROUGH SIXTY   87

MENOPAUSE   92

SIXTY-ONE THROUGH SEVENTY-FIVE   95

SEVENTY-SIX AND OVER   103

    HEARING: 106

    SIGHT: 106

    TASTE AND SMELL: 108

    YOUR MIND: 109

PART ONE

SETTING GOALS

We are all born to be who we are. Your genetic blueprint determines such physical characteristics as eye and hair color, body type, bone structure, height potential and number and distribution of fat cells. Before you are born, most of your physical make-up is set in place. You don't get a vote. Go with it. Do not try to be someone you are not. Why would you want to? Your individuality is what makes you unique. No matter how tall, short, small or large-boned you are, a fit, trim body with good muscle tone is always attractive.

Keep that in mind when you set your fitness goals. Strive for strength, flexibility, cardiovascular endurance and low body fat. Fitness is about optimal health. If you happen to end up looking like a million dollars, that's okay too, isn't it.

Many of us have perceived body imperfections we would like to change. For example, you may tend to carry more weight in one part of the body than you would like. The most common complaints are heavy hips and thighs, heavy mid-sections, and legs that are too thin. You can blame it on the distribution of fat cells in your body. Taking off excess weight and toning can improve, but not significantly change, all of the above.

Now let's explore what many of us perceive as problem areas. We'll start with the hips and thighs. That has been my problem throughout life. I found that doing exercises that tightened the lower hips and thighs (isometrics) improved the muscle tone in that area. My pants fit better now and I'm wearing a smaller size. Weight loss was not necessary for that change.

The mid-section is a concern for both men and women. To flatten the tummy, your best bet is sitting and standing up straight and tightening the abdominal muscles as often as possible. Check for excess fat in that area. You may need to lose some weight in addition to toning.

You say your legs are too thin. You are the envy of many, including me. You may want to try weights to increase muscle bulk. Exercising your legs will develop those muscles and make your legs shapelier.

Do not obsess about being thin. That old saying "you can never be too rich or too thin" is only half-true. Thin is not necessarily fit and fit is not necessarily thin. The tall, willowy, leggy models you see as ideal are the exception, not the rule. Most of us are not meant to be that thin. Striving to be thinner than your body type dictates, can lead to mal-nutrition and serious eating disorders. Don't set yourself up to fail. Keep your goals realistic.

For all you athletes out there: young, not so young, beginners and accomplished. Your goals are strength, flexibility, endurance, technique and coordination. As a swim team coach, I have seen first hand, how an athlete can develop simply by consistent practice and motivation. Many young athletes do not appear to have any special ability when they start, but will suddenly pull ahead of the pack. It is always the result of hard work and determination.

Okay! You have decided it is time for you to get in shape. That's step one. Now, let's explore your options. You need a plan you can live with. In my opinion, exercise is the corner stone of fitness; therefore, your choice of exercise should be something you can enjoy for a minimum of thirty minutes, three to five times per week. Those of you who are strangers to exercise may have to try several types before you find something you don't hate or, hopefully may be fun. (See EXERCISE for details).

Some lifestyle changes will be necessary. Fitness is a way of life. You will need to trade in some of your old habits. Couch potatoes - listen up! Get off that couch and start moving. Don't be surprised if that aerobics class turns out to fun, but beware of those after-class treats with your new friends. If you can't tear yourself away from the group, limit yourself to a cup of coffee or a diet drink. You wouldn't want to cancel out what you've just accomplished.

Setting your ultimate goal is desirable, but short-term goals, when you are on your way, are helpful. Success breeds success. Each time you achieve a plateau, you will be encouraged to continue toward the next one. Along the way, be sure to enjoy every stop.

Today is the day to begin. Do not put it off. As you read this book, I hope you will find all the information you need to achieve your goals. I'll bet you already know most of it.

I wish you all the best on your journey to a fit and healthy life!

Be *YOUR PERSONAL BEST* and you will be a winner. Remember, you are one-of-a-kind.

EXERCISE

When someone asks me what I consider the most important element of a fitness program, without hesitation, my answer is *exercise.* The benefits are enormous. If done at least three times a week for thirty minutes or more, it strengthens the heart, lowers blood pressure, lowers cholesterol, increases HDL cholesterol, and increases the metabolic rate. Oxygen nourishes the brain leading to feeling energetic and alert. Now where can you find a pill that will do all that?

Sorry golfers and bowlers, I know they are fun sports, but they do not qualify as effective exercise. In order to meet your needs for the benefits above, you should include warm-up, stretching, aerobics, strength and flexibility movements and a cool-down. Now don't let that scare you. It's simpler than it sounds.

Before you begin any exercise, you should take a few minutes for mildly stretching the major muscle groups. (Calves, hamstrings, quadriceps, waist, shoulders and arms). Now you're ready for the aerobic segment. Start slowly and gradually increase intensity. Anything that elevates your heart rate, like brisk walking, dancing, swimming, tennis, volleyball etc., for a minimum of twenty minutes, will work. Now that your muscles are warm, it's a good time to do some strength training. Using weights for this portion of your program is beneficial, but not necessary, especially if you are just beginning. Flexing arms, knee bends, leg extensions, lunges and push-ups; anything that works your muscles will increase your strength and build muscle. Remember, muscle burns fat.

You've worked hard. Now it's time to cool down and stretch out. Stretching the major muscle groups at this point is designed for permanent flexibility. Hold each stretch for twenty seconds and repeat three to five times. Never bounce while stretching. Finish your program with foot flexes, ankle rotations, shoulder shrugs and rolls and neck stretches (no neckrolls, please). After two or three deep breaths and slow exhalations, you'll feel totally relaxed. Did I mention that exercise relieves stress?

Exercising on a regular basis should be fun, so pick something you like. If it's boring or just plain drudgery, you won't stick to it - neither would I. Work out with your spouse, the kids or a friend. Here are a few suggestions. Brisk walking is a good way to start out. There are countless videos and records on the market. Be careful not to select one that is too advanced for you. I started out about fourteen years ago, three to four times a week, with a jazzercise record. Before I knew it, I had lost seventeen pounds. Since weight loss was not my goal, I started consuming more calories rather than give up the exercise. I was having too much fun.

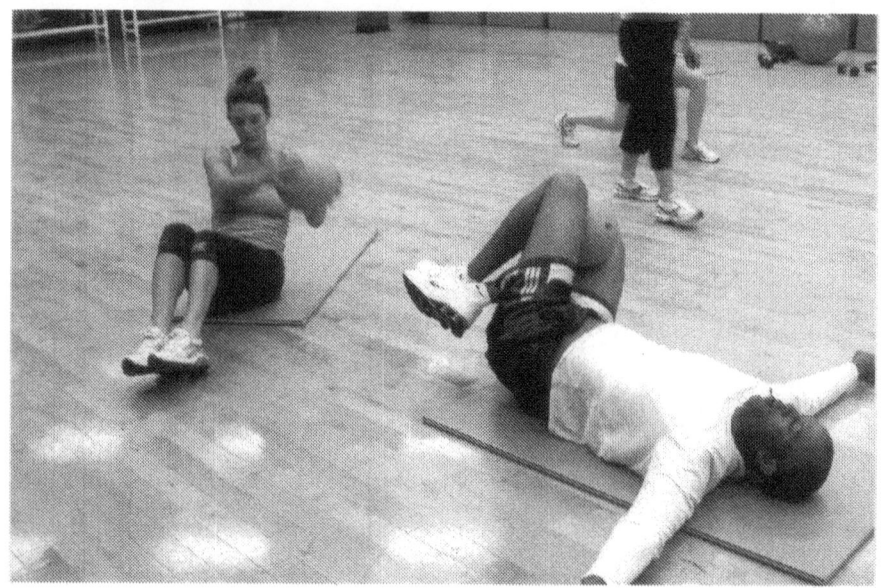

A couple doing floor work at Las Vegas Athletic Club.

Classes are available for aerobics and weight training, both on land and in the water. Before you sign up for any classes, check out the programs and instructors. Make sure the instructors are certified and experienced. Full classes are usually a good indication that the programs are sound.

Most importantly, get started and keep going. You may have to try several different things before you hit on the right activity for you. Don't give up if the first thing you try is not for you. Your choices are endless. Regular exercise is vital to your health and well-being. Make it a priority!

When you have selected your method of exercise, you'll want to improve your fitness level. Progressive overload is the way to go. Extend a little beyond your comfort zone. Work at that level until it becomes comfortable, and then extend again. Proceed with caution. Trying to do too much too soon, can lead to exhaustion and possible injury, not to mention frustration. Perceived exertion is one way to determine if you are working too hard. If you are unable to speak while exercising, you'd better slow down. Be patient. As your fitness level increases, and it will, you will find your heart rate will return to normal more quickly when you stop exercising.

Most beginners, who work out three times per week, can reach a good level of aerobic fitness in twelve weeks. Bear in mind, that fitness cannot be stored. With inactivity, your progress will decline. You should practice progression in all components of fitness: endurance, strength and flexibility.

In your quest for fitness, you need to pay attention to the importance of the mechanics you use when exercising. Proper body alignment is a must - ears over shoulders, shoulders over hips, weight equally distributed on both feet. The human body is designed for movement and, with proper mechanics, it is not likely to break down with use. When there is a deviation from proper postural alignment in one area, there is always a reactive deviation in the opposing muscles.

To stabilize the joints, the muscles supporting the joints must be of equal strength. For example, to support the knee joint properly, the quadriceps (front of the thigh) and hamstrings (back of the thigh) must be of equal strength. All opposing muscles should be equally exercised.

Muscle imbalance is sure to result from poor body alignment (posture) when sitting, standing and walking. Many of us lapse into poor habits without noticing. It's never too late to take stock and make the effort to correct your posture.

ABDOMINALS

As a fitness professional, I am frequently asked advice on what to do about problem areas. Overwhelmingly, the questions involve the abdominals. Reaction to my advice is usually disbelief when I tell them "It's what you do when you're not in exercise class that will flatten your tummy." Here comes that word again - posture. Proper body alignment is necessary to accomplish that goal. I know it sounds old-fashioned, but some things never change.

I'm sure you have seen the quick weight loss commercials with Ms. Before standing with shoulders slumped and lower abdomen protruding in a "let it all hang out" stance. Ms. After, on the other hand, has her shoulders back, her torso held high and her abdomen nicely contracted. Even her legs are positioned together in a more attractive position. She could look ten pounds slimmer without losing an ounce, right? I rest my case.

If you have been walking around for years like Ms. Before, standing and sitting erect will feel unnatural at first. You will only be able to hold your body properly aligned for short periods and still breathe. Don't give up. Do it several times a day whenever you think about it and it will become easier. Do it enough, and it will become second nature. Believe me, your back will thank you and so will your lungs, not to mention the image that looks back at you in the mirror.

You are now sitting and standing up straight, (your second grade teacher would be proud). Let's look at some other things you can do. It you go to an exercise class, contract your abdominals each time you do a squat, step up or down on the step bench, jog in place or perform plies in dance class. As you sit on the stationary bike, see how close you can get your navel to your spine. Don't forget to breathe! If you do all these things, sit-ups and crunches won't be necessary. When improperly done, they can cause back injury, so be sure that you have proper instruction and supervision should you decide to do them. For six-pack abs, you will need weight training and, yes, the dreaded sit-ups and crunches.

You have done all of the above and you see a big improvement. However, there's still a protrusion in the lower abdominal area. The bad news is that it is probably fat. I don't think I need to tell you what to do about that. Weight control is a subject that needs to be dealt with in more detail. We will discuss it further in the Weight Control section.

WEIGHT TRAINING

Want quick results? Head for the weight room. You're sure to see noticeable changes in four to six weeks in the way you look and feel. You'll burn calories, but may not lose much weight at first. Muscle is heavier than fat. However, muscle burns fat and increases metabolic rate, which is the key to weight loss.

A major benefit from weight training is bone health. Bone mass peaks at age twenty to thirty for women. Both men and women begin losing strength, muscle and bone mass after age thirty. The loss occurs so slowly, it's hardly noticeable.

The good news is that middle aged and older adults can gain strength and protect bones at the same rate as younger people do. People who are age sixty and over can improve strength by thirty to one hundred percent.

Why do we want to be strong? For starters, strength and power equal freedom and independence. It enables us to lift, push, and carry things, such as groceries and the kids, upstairs or downstairs. You know - daily living. Your sports performance will be optimal and you will be less vulnerable to injuries. My first encounter with weight training was with a physical therapist who was treating me for a shoulder injury. I was teaching eleven exercise classes per week and training four to five days per week for a national swimming competition. The result? Overuse. Even though I was in good physical condition, I was asking too much of my body. My upper body muscles had to be strengthened. I began my workout with seven minutes on the Nordic Track to warm up. I worked my chest and back muscles and then the triceps and biceps. The goal was toward strength and endurance. To that end, I didn't increase the amount of weight, but rather the number of repetitions and sets. I was amazed at how much stronger my upper body became in the eight weeks I spent with the therapist. However, he did tell me that as long as I kept up my present schedule, I had to continue with the weights for two to three times a week.. To me, that was no hardship. I enjoyed weight training enough to add several additional lower body exercises.

I believe that weight training should be a part of all fitness programs for the above-mentioned reasons. You can train as little as twice a week for forty-five minutes to an hour, as a part of your total exercise program.

I strongly recommend professional guidance, at least starting out. There are classes available at most health clubs. Personal trainers are helpful, but can be pricey when used on a regular basis.

Start out slowly and build in both amount of weight and number of repetitions. Find the weight that stresses you a little. Start out with one set of eight to twelve repetitions. Gradually increase the number of sets until you reach three. Then increase the weight a little. You may have to go back to one or two sets at the heavier weight. Progression is the name of the game.

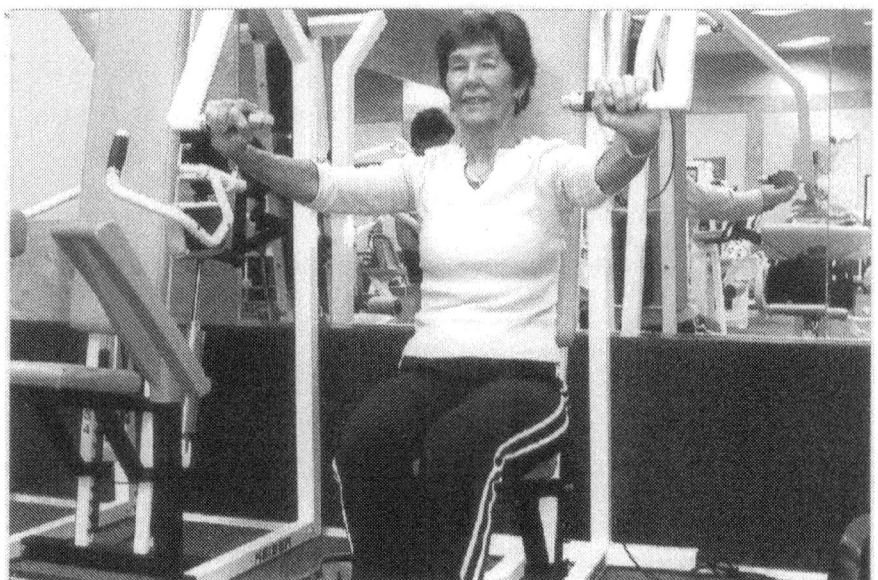

The author working out on the chest press.

WATER EXERCISE

In the past twenty years or so, the fitness industry has been exploring the benefits of exercising in water. In my experience as a water exercise instructor, I have seen water jogging, aqua step, pre-natal water exercise, arthritis exercise, post-operative mastectomy exercise and water aerobics come into their own. From the gentlest to the most vigorous, there is something to suit everyone's needs.

Approximately ninety-five percent of all people enjoy being in water. It is known to be soothing and have therapeutic qualities. Why else would so many of us seek out hot tubs or take a long, hot bath to relax?

The YMCA, The Aquatic exercise Association, and The United States Water Fitness Association are all devoted to promoting excellence in water exercise. All instructors are required to update their certifications every two or three years. Through re-certification, workshops and seminars, instructors are kept abreast of all the latest developments in their field..

People with moderate to severe arthritis can exercise more comfortably and safely in warm water. The muscles, which support the joints, are stretched and strengthened without impact. Many people who need walkers and canes can do without them in water. Simply walking in water can help strengthen leg and arm muscles. Besides, it just plain feels good to those who have difficulty maneuvering on dry land.

When you are waist deep in water, your body weight is reduced to fifty percent; chest deep water brings it down to ten percent. Impact is reduced proportionately.

Recovering from an injury? Deep-water exercise may be for you. Using a flotation device (float belt or bar bells), you can work any part of your body with absolutely no impact. Many runners use this form of exercise as an alternative activity whether they are injured or not. You can actually 'run' up and down the pool without touching the bottom. Your legs will surely know they have worked out.

Water walking is probably the most popular form of water exercise, especially for seniors. The beauty of it is that you can walk or jog at your own level of speed and intensity. Always moving forward, backward or sideways, you can walk slowly, jog, or sprint. The force with which you go through the water will determine the degree of your workout. Here is where water resistance comes into play. For an aerobic workout, running through the water, using both arms and legs will increase your heart rate. Please note that your heart rate will be about ten to twenty beats per minute less than on land with the same amount of exertion. This does not mean that your workout is any less effective. Ankle and wrist weights and mitts, especially designed for use in water, are available for a high intensity workout. Variations of arm and leg movements, such as straight leg raises, knee raises, breaststroke and freestyle arm movements, etc. will add a variety of stretching and contracting to the large muscle groups. Now for the top of the line: A program, which includes aqua-step, water jogging, power moves and deep-water exercise, has it all for a high intensity workout. The resistance of the water produces the same effect as weights. The harder you push against the water, the more resistance you get. Muscle strengthening, toning and an increase in heart rate are the results. This is definitely not for the unfit.

The jury is still out on the question of weight loss. Many experts feel that "burning" calories while your body is being cooled in water, is not as efficient as in land exercise. Not all experts agree.

Bear with me if I get overly enthusiastic about swimming. I've been a swimmer all my life and can't imagine life without it. All of the major muscle groups are worked at once. Add the absence of impact and you have the perfect exercise, right?

For those of you who have minimal swimming skills, they can be easily improved, and a progressive swim schedule will increase your endurance quickly. All you need is a few sessions with a qualified swim instructor or coach. Some feel that swimming laps is boring - not for me. I vary my workout by doing fifty, one hundred or two hundred yard sets of different speeds and strokes. Kick sets with fins and/or a kick board can add more variety.

One of the things I love about swimming is that it is a life-long activity, even if you have difficulty maneuvering on land. I recently participated in a state senior swim meet where I met a ninety-six year old woman who competed. When she completed the race, someone had a walker waiting for her. She beamed as the crowd cheered her. Her waves and facial expression said it all.

I'm proud to say that I swam on the same Masters Swim Team with two remarkable women, who both recently completed the swim across the English Channel, from England to France. In order to qualify for the record book, they had to adhere to the rules set forth by the Channel Swimming Association. There were no wet suits allowed to protect them against the sixty-degree water temperature. The twenty-one mile course is known for its choppy water due to wind and tide. Both women completed the grueling swim in a little more than eleven hours. They are thirty-four and fifty years old. My cap and goggles are off to you, Nancy and Michelle.

Now I'm not suggesting that you aspire to such lofty goals. The pool at the YMCA will do just fine.

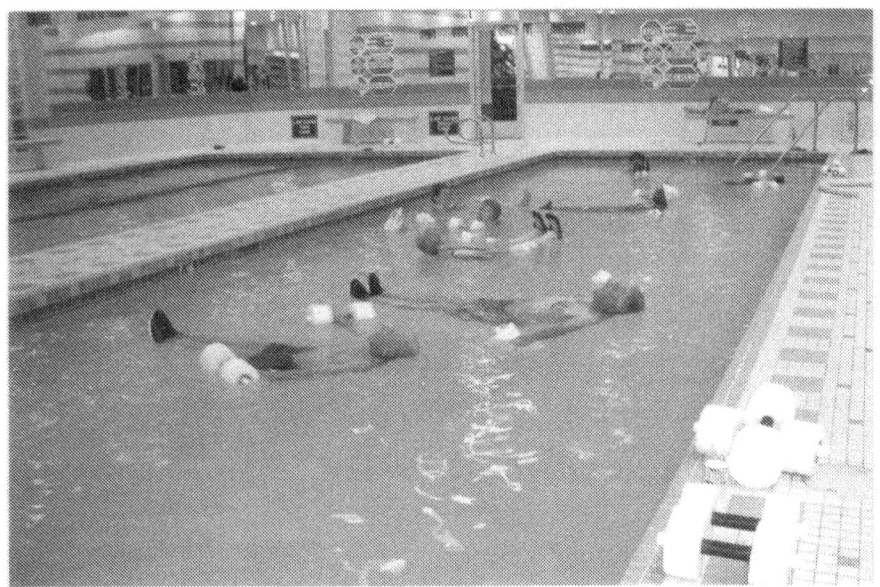

Water exercise is not just for women.

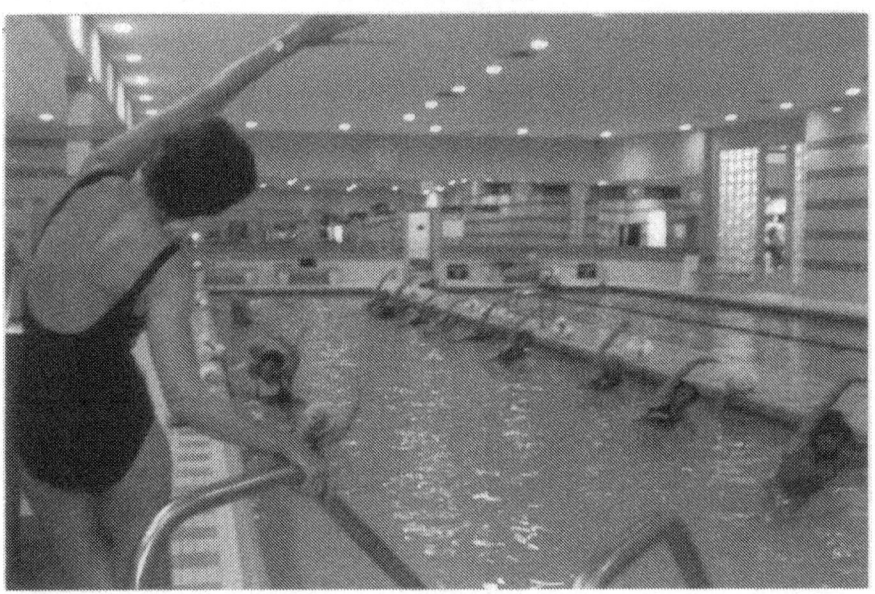

Warm down and stretching

MIND/BODY

The concept of mind/body dates back to ancient times. Yoga has been around for more than five thousand years. I would say that is a good indication of its validity. For optimal health, there must be an integration of the mind, body, spirit and emotions. To quote Christine Northrup, MD, "Not only do our physical organs contain receptor sites for neuro-chemicals of thought and emotion, our organs and immune system can themselves manufacture these same chemicals. What this means is that our entire body feels and expresses emotion - all parts of us "think and feel." White blood cells for instance can produce morphine-like pain relieving substances, and they in turn contain receptor sites for the same substances. So if the ovaries, bowels, and heart make the same chemicals as the brain makes when it thinks, where in the body is the mind. The mind is located throughout the body."

I'm sure you have experienced a physical reaction to anger and fear. Your heart and respiration accelerates. Less obviously, your blood pressure rises. Stress triggers tension headaches and constricted muscles, especially in the neck and shoulders. Your digestion can be disrupted. In time, all of these negative physical reactions can, and will, cause health problems, such as impaired memory, a weakened immune system, high blood pressure, stomach ulcers, skin problems and digestive difficulties. The famous English physician and writer, Jonathan Miller is quoted as saying, "In living things all restlessness is directed toward the achievement of tranquility." To this end, people seek mind/body programs.

Breath is the source of life - a bridge between the body and the mind. Most of us breathe at half of our lung capacity. Deep inhalation and full exhalation, exercises our lungs and increases our lung capacity. Diaphragmatic breathing is the most efficient respiration system. First, breathe through the nose into the belly. Let your stomach expand as you inhale. This is not the time for tightened abs. Still inhaling, bring air into your rib cage area, allowing your ribs to expand sideways. Then fill your upper chest area. Exhale through your mouth in the reverse, until you feel the belly contract, and all air is expelled. Never hold your breath. You'll feel the tension melt away.

Deep breathing, coordinated with slow, controlled movements, is the common thread that connects mind/body techniques.

AI CHI

In the early 1990's, Mr. Jun Konno of Japan added another dimension to mind/body techniques. He created Ai Chi and took it into water. That piqued my attention. My aquatic colleagues and I trained and certified to teach the program. It quickly became one of our most popular classes.

Ai Chi consists of flowing, soft round movements in rhythm with diaphragmatic breathing... Inhale with palms up - exhale with palms down. The inwardly directed focus requires a non-judgmental attention to self. In Ai Chi, we strive not for the precision and rigidity of traditional exercise, but for tranquility.

The postures are performed with shoulders under water and arms resting on the surface. The water temperature must be warm enough to keep the body relaxed (88 to 96 degrees). The warmth of the water enabled my Arthritis students to participate in, and benefit from Ai Chi. The relaxation of the muscles helped them to perform the Arthritis exercises more efficiently and comfortably after an Ai Chi class.

My own experience with Ai Chi was a pleasant surprise. Being as fit as I was, I assumed that my flexibility was at peak. As I went through the postures, I felt every muscle relax and my range of motion grow. An overall feeling of well-being and calm lingered long after the class ended. Now, I do Ai Chi almost every day, even when I'm not teaching.

One more thing I feel is worthy of mention. I had a student with Muscular Dystrophy, who used a walker and wore braces on her legs. She was able to get into the water without any of those devices and perform all of the postures with ease. Her range of motion was huge. Doing Ai Chi was a joy for her.

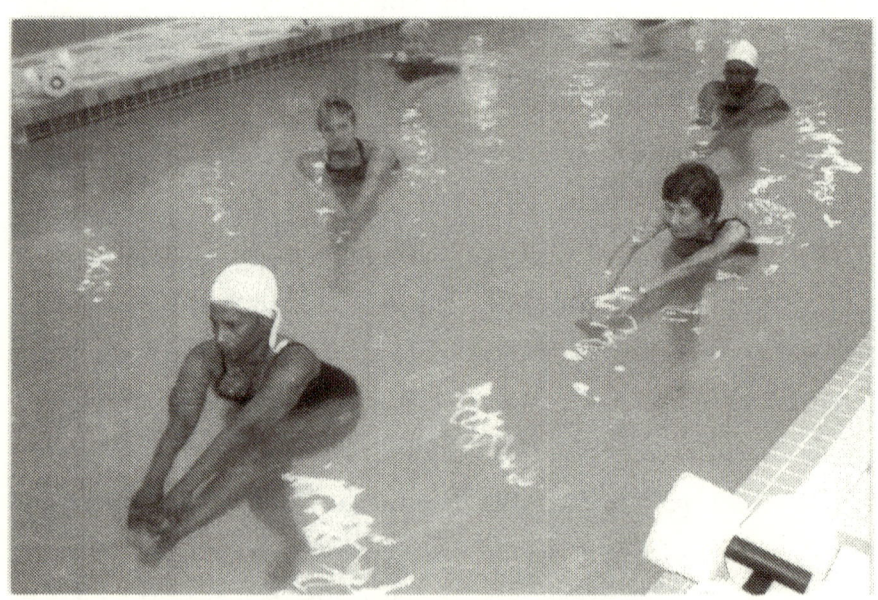

Ai Chi Posture – rounding

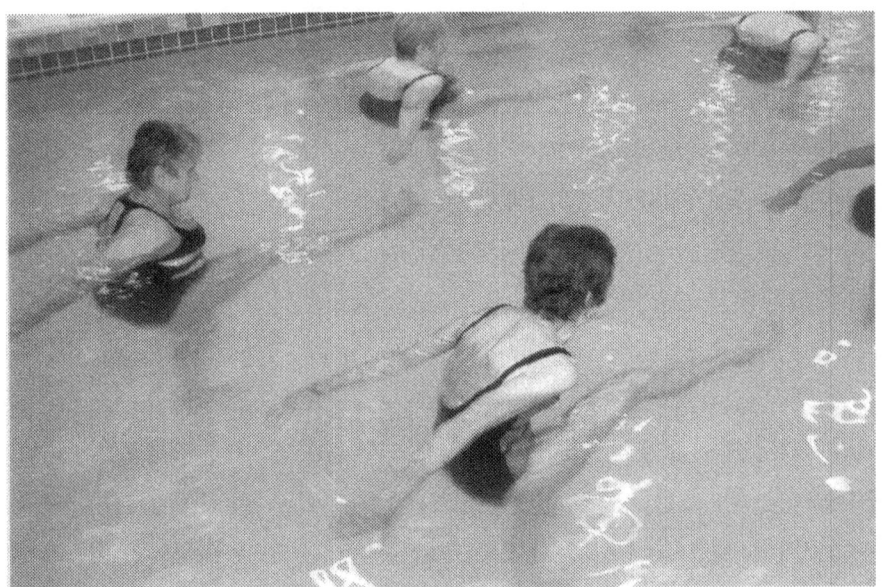

Ai Chi Posture – balancing

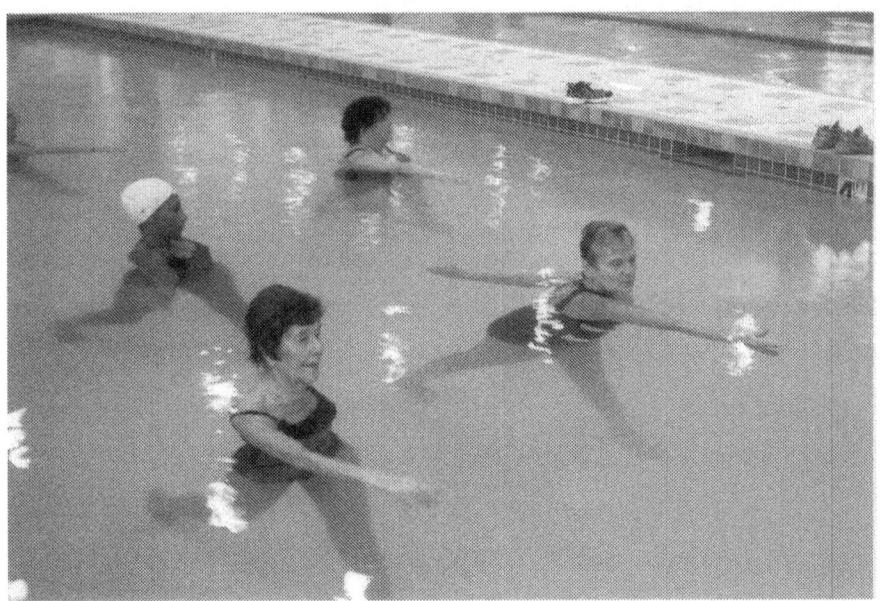

Ai Chi Posture – gathering

PILATES

Pilates was developed during the confinement of a German in an English internment camp during World War I. His desire to help patients rehabilitate while lying in bed, led him to rig springs above the beds. This setup later evolved into one of the main pieces of equipment in the Pilates method. His name - Joe Pilates.

He immigrated to the United States in 1923 and opened a studio on 8th Avenue in New York City. He began training and rehabilitating professional dancers. Today, Pilates is one of the most popular exercises in American health clubs. Originally called Contrology, it was developed to build abdominal strength and body control. It is excellent for rehabilitation of the back, knee, hip, shoulders and repetitive stress injuries.

Mental focus and deep breathing are the cornerstones of the program. There are specific breathing cues for every exercise. Pull navel to spine is the first ultimate Pilates cue.

Strengthening the body core (mainly abdominals), lengthening the spine, building muscle tone and increasing body awareness and flexibility, are all goals of Pilates. It teaches how to focus on the muscle being worked, while relaxing all others.

Make no mistake - Pilates is not easy, but the results are worth it. If you are a novice, begin with pre-Pilates.

One of the most unlikely enthusiasts of Pilates is one of my Arthritis students. She is seriously impaired by the disease and suffers a great deal of pain and restriction of movement. Since I viewed Pilates as a strength and power program, I never would have recommended it for her. However, the combination of the Arthritis Aquatic Program and Pilates is working wonders for her.

TAI CHI

It is generally agreed among historians that Tai Chi was developed in the Sung Dynasty (960-1279 A.D.), by the famous boxer Chang San-feng. Somewhat related to Chinese boxing, it is an art of self-defense and physical exercise based on effortless breathing, rhythmic movement and equilibrium. The essence of Tai Chi lies in the maintenance of perfect body balance at all times. The lower the center of gravity, and the larger its base, the greater its stability. For this reason, Tai Chi movements are executed in a semi-crouched position.

The technique is comprised of 128 movements, which can be reduced to 37, by eliminating repetitions and preserving the essential ones. Once properly learned, it is possible to run through the simplified course of 37 movements in three to five minutes.

Deeply rooted in Chinese philosophy, which, admittedly, I do not completely understand, I will attempt to define it more clearly by the principles as set forth by the Tai Chi masters:

"In any action, the whole body must be made as light and free-moving as possible."

Yuan: **Make your motions in a circular way, thus aiming for internal and external harmony**

Sung: **Relax both inside and outside to promote blood circulation**

Ching: **Do not tense your body or become rigid, so that you may be able to move lightly**

Yun: **Move at an even speed controlled by your mind**

Cheng: **Maintain good balance and posture, not letting the body lean to either side**

Shu: **Move your body in an easy, comfortable and relaxed way**

Tsing: **Drive out worldly thoughts from the mind and concentrate your mind.**

Tai Chi aims for total relaxation of the body and perfect balance vs. weight, force and speed.

Introduced to the western world around the 1960's, Tai Chi has gained popularity in the United States. It is suitable for all ages. Seniors flock to Tai Chi classes.

YOGA

As I mentioned earlier, Yoga has been in existence for more than five thousand years. It has been widely practiced by Americans as far back as I can remember and gaining in popularity. Yoga studios are popping up all over the country. Meditation, along with deep breathing and controlled movements, are the components that are contained in Yoga techniques. It teaches you to quiet the mind and relax the body.

Meditation evokes the full relaxation response, thus achieving a deep sense of calm. Blood pressure drops, heart and respiration rates slow and the muscles become less tense.

The medical profession is beginning to pay attention to what Yoga practitioners have known for a long time. The mind can destroy health with negative thoughts, such as stress, fear, hostility, hopelessness. On the other hand, the mind has healing powers. Yoga devotees will attest to that. One woman told me that she controls her diabetes with Yoga. Countless people believe wholeheartedly in the health benefits of practicing Yoga. From weight control to pain management, Yoga is the choice of many.

The relaxed state achieved during Yoga exercises, allows the body to attain maximum flexibility. My daughter, an exercise physiologist, loves Yoga because, aside from the health benefits, the graceful rhythmic movements are reminiscent of her beloved ballet.

Yoga is many things to many people, most of whom view it as their lifeline. A few people commented that mind-body exercises are not vigorous enough for them. I say, "Don't knock it until you've tried it." The lack of cardio-vascular does not make it an ineffective exercise. Aside from the soothing relaxation, there are very real benefits, such as strength and flexibility, to gain. Learning to exercise in a state of total relaxation is an important factor in your overall quest for fitness.

SPORTS/DANCE

Tennis anyone? How about softball, volleyball, basketball, track and field and all the others? Time was, once your school days were over, so were your sports - not so anymore. I remember someone telling me to "act your age" when I was belly flopping down a snow-covered hill with my toddler. I was 26! When I reached 30, I thought I was getting too old for water skiing. Thank God! We now realize that age doesn't slow us up unless we allow it to happen. Professional athletes are enjoying careers that extend far beyond what was once thought possible.

Now there are endless outlets for athletes of all ages. Competitive or non-competitive, YMCA's, communities and masters programs offer a variety of sports where you can participate with others your own age. Don't let the word "masters" scare you. It simply means that you are nineteen or older and are not competing scholastically. Some of my adult "learn to swim" students, went directly to the Masters Swim Team, as soon as they could complete fifty yards. Not only did they find a great fitness regime, they made new friends and had a great time.

Most of us participated in one sport or another in school. Why not pick up where you left off or try something new? Chances are, you could add a completely new dimension to your life!

Dancing is another activity we tend to abandon once we leave our teens. There are many varieties of adult dance classes available. To name a few: ballroom, tap, ballet, and line dancing. Country line dancing is my favorite. I simply pop a tape into the VCR and dance along.

Whatever activity you choose, do it consistently, two or three times a week. Whether alone, with a friend or family member, or in a group, have fun. You'll find your spirit will rise and, just maybe, your waistline will diminish.

WEIGHT CONTROL/DIET

You are reading this book because you have decided to get fit. For some of you, that may mean losing weight. Your first impulse will probably be to look for a quick fix. Resist the temptation.

Let's look at some of the fad diets from the past. In 1967, there was the *Stillman Quick Weight Loss Diet*. Dr. Stillman advocated a very low-carbohydrate, high-protein diet consisting of mainly cottage cheese, eggs, seafood, poultry, and meat. The diet virtually forbade fruits, vegetables and grain foods.

Dr. Atkins Diet Revolution, another low-carbohydrate plan, burst upon the diet scene in 1972. It allowed you to eat just about all of the fat you wanted. Then came the *Scarsdale Diet* in 1978 - another low-carbohydrate, high-protein plan. People lost weight on the diets, but a lot of it was water weight. There were some unhealthy side effects. Most people found it impossible to stay on such diets, gave up, and quickly regained the weight.

In 1981, came the introduction of the *Cambridge Diet*, which became widely adopted. It consisted of only liquid in the form of a couple of protein-rich drinks a day, totaling 320 calories. Health problems resulted. A good friend of mine had to be hospitalized after being on this diet for three weeks. I could continue with many other examples, but I think I made my point. DIETS JUST DO NOT WORK!

The notion that weight gain is inevitable with aging is something I refuse to believe. What I do believe is that we have more control over our weight and physical condition than we want to take responsibility for. I'm sure there are many people who have eating disorders due to deep psychological problems. Most of us, however, have simply fallen into poor eating habits and all too sedentary life styles.

At this point, I'd like to share with you my own experience with a weight problem. It happened very suddenly. When I returned to school after summer vacation to start my junior year in high school, I realized I was overweight. I tried to control my sweet tooth, but I just couldn't. It wasn't until I was eighteen years old and working in an office, that I finally faced the fact that I was overweight because I was eating high calorie food. Having tried diets and failed, I made up my mind to change my eating habits permanently. It was surprisingly simple. I ate the same breakfast I had always eaten: orange juice, cereal and coffee. For lunch, I substituted a bowl of soup and some crackers for the large sandwich and equally large wedge of layer cake I had been eating. Dinner was whatever Mom put on the table, but the two slices of bread and butter had to go, along with dessert. I checked my habit to go for a second helping. I found out I really didn't need it. I've never been big on total self-denial, so occasionally I'd have a snack at night. Also, I allowed myself ice cream or pizza (small) when I was out with my friends. Two months later, without really dwelling on it, I had lost twenty pounds. I was satisfied with the way I looked and felt.

That is not the end of the story. It has worked for me for sixty years-through the birth of two children, menopause, into my golden years. My weight is the same as it was when I lost those twenty pounds.

I made a choice, which enabled me to live a better quality of life. I still have a sweet tooth that won't quit, but it's under control. I find I can have my sweets in limited quantities and still maintain low body fat. You can too.

Let's face it! Food high in fat and sugar tastes good. The thought of giving up cheeseburgers, fries, pizza, ice cream, etc. can be depressing. If you eat sensibly every day and save the "forbidden" foods for a once-in-a-while treat, in limited quantities, you can accomplish permanent weight control. It's your choice.

I am not a nutritionist. Not many of us are. Unless you have been living in a cave, cut off from the world at large, you already know which foods are healthy and which cause unwanted weight gain. Just about every day, you'll read or hear, on television, in newspapers and magazines and in school, all of the nutritional facts you need to plan a healthy diet. Here's where common sense comes into play. I don't need to provide you with a food pyramid, illustrating what percentage of each food group you need each day. It seems that changes almost daily. Who is going to figure it out anyway?

I realize that many of you need to lose more than the twenty pounds I took off in my teens. Some of you may need guidance. *Weight Watchers* is the only program I know of, that can teach you to permanently change your eating habits and, at the same time, offer you a support group. They have a history of success stories of people who have taken off weight and kept it off. Many other factors play a part in weight control. Exercise is a must when you are losing weight. Without it, you will lose both fat *and* muscle. Building muscle while you are losing weight is essential.

Never underestimate that magnificent machine we call the human body. Among other miraculous functions, your body self-adjusts. If you subject it to long periods without food, it will conserve fuel by slowing down the fuel burning process (metabolism) and store calories in the form of fat. Not exactly what you had in mind when you decided to skip breakfast or any other meal, right?

Your metabolic rate is largely predetermined by heredity, sex (women have a slower rate than men) and your age. While it's true that some of us have a naturally speedy metabolism, don't make the mistake of simply accepting the fact that yours is slow and you're stuck with it. *When* you eat, has a profound effect on your metabolic rate.

Skipping breakfast is rapidly becoming an American way of life for today's busy families. Who has time to sit down and eat in the morning? When you realize the adverse effects that skipping a meal can have on your body, I'm sure you'll agree that taking ten to fifteen minutes in the morning to eat is well worth it. If you are really pressed for time, a glass of fruit juice or a piece of fruit, a non-sugar coated cold cereal with low-fat milk (no pastries, please) and a hot drink take no preparation time, and virtually no clean-up is required. Not only will you get your metabolism going, but your energy level will become more constant. I'll even go one-step further and recommend low-fat snacks at regular intervals. Your metabolic rate will increase and you will not be tempted to eat everything in sight at dinnertime.

The alarming epidemic of obesity in the United States is partially a result of our American Culture, which dictates that we eat our major meal late in the day. Physical activity after dinner is unlikely, causing the fats and carbs consumed during that large meal, to be stored in the body as fat if they are not used.

Your metabolism rate changes throughout the day, and is slowest when you are asleep. Eating breakfast will wake it up. Exercise, especially aerobic and weight training, revs up your metabolism; and will keep it at a higher level for hours after you have stopped.

What does food mean to you? Aside from sustaining life, enjoying a meal with family and friends, is a great way to interact with others. Sharing dinner with the family can be a time for us to reconnect at the end of the day. Celebrations, holidays and parties all revolve around food and drink. By the way, alcoholic beverages and soft drinks are usually high in calories and we tend not to count liquids when we are assessing our caloric intake. Many of our favorite foods are reserved for a special occasion. For example, served for Thanksgiving we have turkey and all the trimmings. Here is where we can get into trouble. Of course, you don't want to miss any of those rare culinary treats. Who can blame you - certainly not me. I'm with you. The trick is moderation. I discovered quite a few years ago that I could enjoy everything on the Thanksgiving menu without stuffing myself. Only the turkey should be stuffed. I have also learned that the uncomfortable feeling following overeating ruined my ability to enjoy the rest of the party.

Extra calories on special occasions will not significantly shoot down your fitness level, especially if there is no interruption in your exercise regime. You can relax and enjoy your holidays guilt-free.

Even if your eating and drinking do get a little out of control during a party, don't despair. Nobody is perfect.

Dining out? Is it necessary to forego your favorite entree because it's calorie laden? Not necessarily - ask your waiter to bring you a box with the entree. Cut the serving in half and place the other half in the box. It's not only what you eat, but how much.

Now let's look at some of the other pitfalls of dining out. Appetizers are usually high in calories and certainly not essential to the enjoyment of a good meal. The salad bar usually offers a variety of dishes that can also be high in calories. Avoid the ones prepared with mayonnaise and fat-laden dressings. A combination of lettuce, tomatoes and raw carrots, dressed with vinegar and oil, will satisfy your desire for salad.

Now, about dessert - have you had a cocktail or two? If so, dessert is a no, no. Make a choice; if you have eaten at a leisurely pace, you should be feeling full and satisfied by the end of the meal.

Some of us eat when we are not hungry. Emotional reasons such as boredom, loneliness, disappointment, depression and stress can cause us to eat to make ourselves feel better; but it seldom does. Guilt often follows, thus creating a vicious cycle. It is within your power to break that cycle. Find something else to substitute for that behavior. Take a walk, make a phone call, clean out a drawer, take the dog out - anything that will distract you until you get over the urge. Self-discipline will be required until you get beyond the habit of emotional eating. Structuring your eating times will help. Schedule your snacks. I know it sounds dreary, but if you are determined to get and stay fit, eliminating habits such as this, is necessary. Is it worth it? Most definitely!

Adequate hydration is essential to weight control, as well as to general good health. You must have heard of the recommended eight glasses of water per day. Why? Dehydration can cause decreased physiological function, including the process of fat metabolism. When you are dehydrated, your body goes in search of water, which can cause you to eat when you are not actually hungry. It's a good idea to drink a glass of water about a half-hour before a meal. Not only will your stomach feel full, the water will also help your digestive system function more efficiently.

Can we count liquids other than plain water? Not really - carbonated and caffeinated beverages have a diuretic effect, causing your body to lose water.

Drink water *before* you feel thirsty. By that time, chances are you are already dehydrated. Adequate hydration during exercise will keep you body cool and energized.

When it comes to your ideal weight, do not make the mistake of picking a number out of the air. The important thing is the ratio of lean body mass to body fat. For women, eighteen to twenty-five percent is the norm. It is normal for men to have less body fat than women. They can go as low as eight percent and still fall into the normal range. You can have your body fat measured, but I believe you will know when you have reached a good weight.

The worldwide epidemic of obesity is alarming. What is even more alarming, is that it is affecting more and more children. More than fifty-percent of adults in the United States are overweight. Genes do play a part in obesity; but the bottom line is excess weight is the result of taking in more calories than you burn.

If you are not vigilant, creeping weight gain happens to adults starting around age twenty-five. Here's how it happens. You gain between five and ten pounds a year - no big deal, right. You still can wear the same size clothing and you really don't look fat. You reason that you are getting older and a little weight gain is normal. Wait a minute! Aren't you in control? If you permit a weight gain of five pounds per year, in ten years you will have gained fifty pounds! It was so gradual, that you hardly noticed; but fifty pounds, you do!

Suppose you checked that first five-pound gain. In order to do that, you need to cut a few calories (it doesn't take much), and get a little more exercise. I guarantee that ten years down the road life will be better for you.

Let's not make weight control any more complicated than it is. There are no secrets, or magic formulas, that will stabilize your weight. The formula is simple - calories ingested vs. calories burned, with the above-mentioned factors in the mix.

Old habits die hard. How determined are you to stabilize your weight and fitness level? You have a lot at stake: your health, appearance and self-esteem. Eat wisely and enjoy every day of your life!

AGING

We begin aging the moment we are born. From that day forward, for the next eighty or ninety years or more, we will undergo thousands of physical and mental changes. We will grow, develop and eventually, deteriorate. How we age, and the rate at which we age, is impacted by our genetic makeup, some of which, we can do little about. More significantly, our lifestyle strongly influences the aging process; the food we do, or do not eat, our experiences, how we think or feel and, more importantly, how we act upon those processes, will affect the rest of our lives.

The first visible signs of aging appear on the skin in the early thirties. That is when you will notice the faint beginnings of lines and wrinkles. As in most physical characteristics, your genetic make-up essentially determines how your skin ages. How you care for your skin plays an equally significant role in your appearance. Sun damage, smoking, stress, lack of sleep and drug use can have an adverse effect on your skin.

Let's look at the important role your body's largest organ (your skin) plays in your overall health. Without your skin to protect you, your blood, lymph, water and other life-sustaining fluids, would evaporate. You would have no defense against ultraviolet rays. Your skin also acts as your immune system's front-line defense. In addition, your skin produces perspiration, which regulates body temperature and allows your blood vessels to dilate; thus releasing body heat.

I'm not going to tell you how to keep your skin looking young. I'll leave that to the plastic surgeons, dermatologists and beauty experts. My concern is for the health of the skin. We all know that the sun can damage your skin. We fortify ourselves with sunscreen in the summer when we know we'll be spending all day outdoors. That's fine, but the sun can cause damage all year around. That's why you must protect your skin at all times. You can even sustain sun damage while driving your car. I'm certainly not a person who uses many cosmetics, but all of my moisturizers and foundations contain anywhere from SPF 6 through SPF 15. Speaking of moisturizers, regular use helps relieve dryness and minimizes the appearance of fine lines and wrinkles. Don't forget your sunglasses any time you are exposed to the sun; winter, summer, spring and fall. They will not only protect your eyes, but also help to prevent those "squint" lines around your eyes. Gentlemen: you are not immune.

Skin cancer is more common than we would like to believe. I have watched my sister, my daughter and two of my friends go through the treatment. All required surgery. Why risk it? It can kill you.

Healthy bone growth begins in early childhood and peaks at age twenty to thirty. Unless you take steps to avoid it, you are at risk for osteoporosis in your declining years. Small, thin-boned men and women are at higher risk. Postmenopausal women may lose bone mass due to the loss of estrogen. You can counteract bone loss by limiting the use of alcohol, tobacco, caffeine and eating calcium-rich food. Weight bearing exercises are beneficial. (See Weight Training)

Good nutrition, plenty of exercise, lots of rest, normal weight level, and lack of stress and a good outlook on life are all components of a healthy life style.

You're probably not thinking about what's down the road for you, while you're trying to manage a job, kids and the mortgage payments. Some days, your objective is just to get through the day. I know. I've been there. The best advice I can give you is to make enough time for yourself to stay fit. You need it. You deserve it. Keep in mind, it is easier to stay fit than to get fit.

As we age, our cardio respiratory capacity, muscle mass, and flexibility diminish at approximately one percent per year from age thirty to sixty-five, then it accelerates to two percent. Don't tell that to the fifty-year-old woman who completed the grueling swim across the English Channel in record time in August of 2004. The fact is that 50% of age-related loss of function is due to inactivity rather than to the aging process.

I experienced a noticeable difference when I reached seventy. It seemed I couldn't swim as fast as I did in the previous ten years but I could still out-swim many master swimmers in their forties and fifties.

Staying active cannot stop the aging process, but it can slow it down considerably. The older we get the more we need to keep moving. It's never too late to make good choices in diet and exercise. Although many experts believe that our life span is genetically determined, leading research authorities also believe that up to 2/3 of all deaths can be attributed to lifestyle choices.

Physical abilities such as coordination, balance, strength and flexibility are crucial to leading an independent life. Isn't that what we all want? Regular exercise will help maintain your fitness level so that you are able to perform the simple tasks required in everyday living. It will also aid in weight control. That arthritic knee would not be so painful if it didn't have to bear more weight than it was meant to.

Many older adults are living with chronic diseases such as arthritis, diabetes, high blood pressure and cardiovascular problems. I'm sure your doctor will agree that it is vital to your health to remain active. Water exercise offers a number of good programs for people with chronic health problems. Simply taking a walk a few days a week can increase your fitness level. Make sure to consult your doctor before embarking on any exercise program.

The importance of flexibility is highly underrated. It will decrease rapidly if your muscles are not stretched on a regular basis. Nothing ages you faster than the inability to move freely. Your range of motion becomes smaller and the demands of everyday living become more difficult. It requires very little time and effort to remain agile well into your seventies and beyond. All it takes is stretching on a regular basis. Take a lesson from your pet. Doesn't he/she stretch several times per day?

Aging is a natural process. Keeping a healthy mental outlook is just as important as staying physically active. Learning new tasks will take a little more time than it used to. Don't let that discourage you. For example, so many seniors, including me, are learning to deal with computers. I'm still in the learning process and probably will be for quite some time. It has opened up a completely new world for me. It was necessary for me to learn in order to write this book. For that, I am grateful.

We have years of experiences which we can apply to new adventures. This age of technology we are living in offers endless exciting possibilities. The choice is yours.

Take advantage of it! Enjoy!

ARTHRITIS

Got twinges in your hinges? Chances are that you are one of the forty-three million Americans suffering from some kind of arthritis, two hundred and fifty thousand of whom are under eighteen years old. By the time we reach forty years of age, nine out of ten of us will have a touch of arthritis, but probably will not be aware of it. The effects of arthritis may range from minor pain, swelling and stiffness to total disability.

Since most forms of arthritis affect the joints, we need to understand a bit about them. Our bodies contain nearly one hundred fifty joints, allowing us the wide range of movement most of us take for granted. When arthritis affects one or more of those joints, it often results in pain, which can lead to restricted movement.

Joints are formed where two or more bones meet. Cartilage, a tough rubbery tissue, covers the ends of the bones, acting as a shock absorber and allowing smooth movement. The joint capsule is the outer shell, enclosing all of the components, which make up the joint. The synovial membrane lines the capsule and secretes synovial fluid. Its job is to lubricate the joints. Muscles, tendons and ligaments surround and support your joints. The bursa, a small sac located near the joint, but is not part of it, serves to cushion the area between bones, tendons and muscles.

There are more than one hundred forms of arthritis. The most common variety is osteoarthritis (OA), which most of us associate with aging. Though it is true that aging is a factor, many people (12.1 percent), as young as twenty-five, have symptoms of OA.

Genetics can play a role in developing OA. For example, people who are born with bowed legs or knock-knees can develop OA due to improper joint alignment.

Joint injuries, which change the stability or alignment of the joint, can result in irregular wear, which in turn, can lead to OA.

OA usually affects the weight-bearing joints such as knees, hips and spine. Stress on the joint causes a breakdown of the cartilage, and sometimes bone (wear and tear), resulting in osteoarthritis. Excess weight puts stress on knees and hips, contributing to OA. When we are young and healthy, cartilage rebuilds itself, but eventually, we break down more than we can build.

The second most common variety is rheumatoid arthritis (RA). It is a serious disease, which left untreated, can damage your joints and lead to complications in other parts of your body. An autoimmune disease, it can affect the covering of the heart, small blood vessels, lungs, eyes, mouth, lymph glands, or spleen. It causes your body to attack itself. The cause is unknown. Some researchers believe a virus triggers it.

I am inclined to believe that theory because I am unlucky enough to have contracted it. It came on suddenly - without warning. I went to bed one night and awakened in the morning with agonizing pain in both hands. I could not move them. After about five minutes, I could move my fingers slightly. I could not hold a toothbrush or grip anything else. Alarmed, I rushed to my doctor, who immediately took a blood test, which revealed an extremely high rate of inflammation in my blood. The rheumatologist, to whom he sent me, came up with a diagnosis of rheumatoid arthritis. He treated me aggressively with high doses of steroids. The year following that diagnosis, was the worst of my life. So far, I have been lucky. I am off all drugs and relatively pain free. The doctor told me I could have another flare-up at any time - so far, so good. Oddly enough, this is a frequent occurrence for the onset of RA. Following the initial onset, RA may take any number of paths, ranging from complete remission to a lifetime of disability.

Lupus, like rheumatoid arthritis, is another serious autoimmune disease. It usually affects women between the ages of fifteen and forty. The symptoms include aching joints, fever and rashes. Sometimes a distinctive butterfly-shaped rash across the cheeks and nose may appear upon exposure to the sun. Fatigue, weight loss, lethargy and lack of appetite, as well as hair loss may also occur. In severe cases, there may be inflammation or swelling of the lining around the heart, lungs, or abdomen. Heart failure can occur if the inflammation is not treated.

In Fibromyalgia, the muscles, ligaments and tendons, rather than the joints, are affected. It is found in women more often than men, and usually occurs between the ages of twenty and fifty. It is difficult to diagnose. There are no definitive blood tests or x-rays to confirm the diagnosis. The doctor must rely on symptoms, which include pain and stiffness, usually in the neck, shoulders, hips and lower back. Many experience severe fatigue. Other symptoms include headaches, irritable bowel syndrome, abdominal pain, constipation or diarrhea. Sleep disorders and restless leg movements, depression or anxiety are common complaints. Having no energy and a lot of pain, the last thing a person suffering with fibromyalgia feels like doing is exercising. However, exercise can be an effective treatment. Walking or water exercise can be a good starting point. Begin slowly and work up to longer and faster periods.

I have touched on some of the most common forms of arthritis. A wealth of information exists in libraries and on the Internet for anyone wishing to pursue the subject further.

Okay. You suspect you may have arthritis. You know there is no cure, and it is sometimes degenerative and even disabling. What do you do now? Run, (if you can) do not walk, to a good rheumatologist. Medication can control the inflammation and pain. He/she may also prescribe physical therapy or a regular exercise program. The Arthritis Foundation and your local YMCA can both meet your needs.

Daily exercise and stretching are an absolute must. Many people find that pain and stiffness are most severe in the early morning. Why not do some mild stretches while you are still in bed? It'll get you going. Stretching in the shower is another option. The warm water will loosen your joints and muscles. Daily exercise can accomplish increased mobility, flexibility, muscle strength and less pain. Warm water exercise is a good place to start. That wonderful feeling of weightlessness in the water makes it easier to move the joints. Many people are able to accomplish movements in water that they cannot do on land.

Swimming, walking and stationary biking (with little or no tension) can all build muscle without stress on the joints. Working with light weights, under professional supervision, can also help you reach your goal to strengthen the muscles, which support the joints, increase range of motion and develop endurance.

Listen to what your body is telling you. If you should feel pain for more than two hours after you have exercised, it is likely that you overdid it. Some muscle soreness is normal after exercising, but pain is not. You will most likely have good and bad days. Modify your exercises during a flare-up or on days when you are experiencing more pain than usual. Try not to stop your routine altogether.

Many claims have been made that certain foods or special diets can relieve or alleviate the discomfort of arthritis. So far, there is no scientific proof to back up those claims. However, a good, nutritious, well-balanced diet will benefit your general good health. Excess weight will put pressure on the knee and hip joints. You may need to lower your caloric intake if you are overweight.

Your mental outlook can make or break your treatment. Depression, anxiety and loss of confidence and self-esteem are common. This is where you are in control. Make a commitment to be the best that you can be. Keep active mentally, physically and socially. Distract yourself from pain with projects that you enjoy and can handle. Focus on what you can do, rather than what you cannot. Fatigue is common for people with arthritis. Be sure to get plenty of rest.

The students in my arthritis exercise classes are outstanding examples of 'positive mental attitude and commitment'. They come to class faithfully no matter what, some using canes and walkers. Many have had joint replacements and have returned to class as soon as they were able. For them, it is just as much a social experience as it is an exercise class. Numbering about thirty, we used to go out for lunch once a month. We gave our senior member a surprise birthday party for his 90th. He is the darling of the group. He lights up the pool with his sunny disposition. These people truly care about each other. Although they have been together for years, each new member is welcomed with genuine warmth and acceptance. This is not only an exercise class; it is a social event where they can go to enjoy a few laughs with friends.

You may wonder why I included a section about arthritis in this book. The answer to that is eventually, most of you will have to deal with the disease. It's a fact. The good news is that it is usually manageable. With proper medication and daily exercise, you can enjoy a better quality of life.

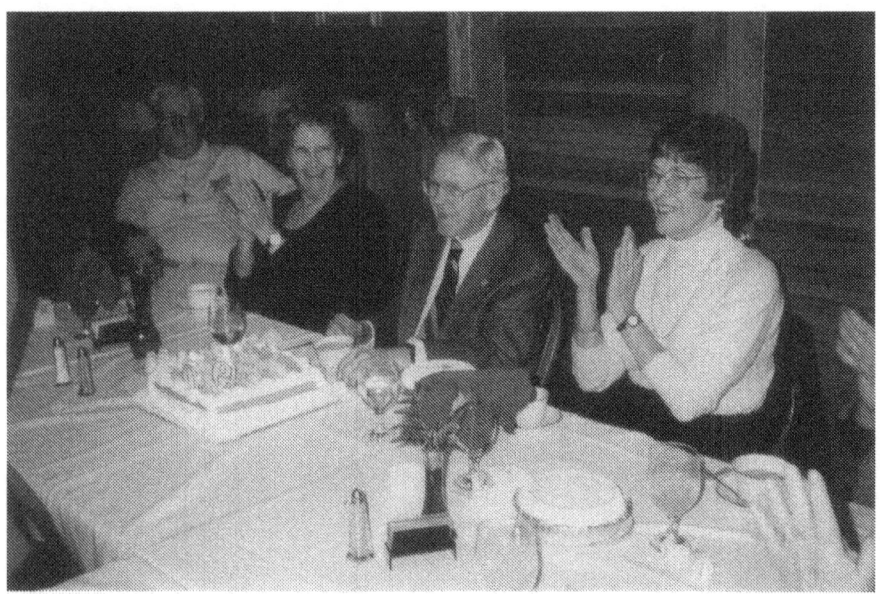

Oscar Benson (second from right), enjoying his ninetieth birthday party.

OSTEOPOROSIS

You probably hear the word osteoporosis (literally means porous bones), on a daily basis. When it comes to senior health, eventually, a doctor will recommend a bone density test, especially if the patient is shrinking in height. The fact is that forty percent of women and ten percent of men will develop osteoporosis. It can be a serious disease, even fatal; however, there is much you can do to prevent bone loss.

Thin, porous bones can lead to fractures. Compression fractures of the vertebrae are the most common cause of loss of height. In most cases, we are unaware that they are happening. Persistent back pain could be the only symptom. Dowager's hump and/or spinal deformities may result. The skeletal structure changes can affect your abdominal organs. Decreased appetite, weight loss, constipation and a protruding belly could follow. If you find yourself short of breath, you may have had compression fractures in the thoracic spine, which could affect your lung expansion.

We seem to hear a lot about elderly people falling and breaking a hip. Actually, the fracture occurs in the femur, which is connected to the pelvis. Most likely, the fracture caused the fall - not the other way around. Unfortunately, there is a twenty percent fatality rate within a year of the injury. Another twenty percent will require confinement to a nursing home within a year of the injury. It happened to both my mother and my grandmother.

Anyone with osteoporosis needs to be especially careful to avoid falls. There are many reasons why older people fall, such as: dizziness, hearing problems, multiple medications, confusion, poor balance, arthritis pain, and poor eyesight. You would be wise to make some changes in your home that could prevent you from falling. I love my 'handicapped' shower, which has two seats and grab bars. I don't use the seats, but I do use the grab bars. It's not something I would have opted for, given a choice, but I am glad that I have it.

Freeing your home from clutter, especially on stairs and floors, will give you less chance for tripping. Your slippers should be non-skid. I rarely wear regular shoes in the house, but stocking feet are not an option for me - too slippery. Even non-skid throw rugs can present a hazard. They can still slide on a highly waxed floor, or you could trip on the edge of the rug. When you use the stairs, make sure you use the handrail. Avoid carrying large loads up and down stairs. When getting out of bed, or up from a chair, do it slowly, and make sure you have your balance before starting to walk. Adequate lighting in your home can prevent accidents.

Women build bone until they reach age thirty to thirty-five. After that, bones begin to lose density unless we take steps to prevent it. Hopefully, when you were growing up, you had a calcium-rich diet and got plenty of weight-bearing exercise, such as walking, running, jumping and anything else that defies gravity.

Men develop more bone mass than women merely because they have more testosterone, which stimulates bone growth and maintains their strength. Osteoporosis does not affect men for ten or more years later than women. By the time men reach age eighty-six, the risk factor becomes even with women. While women experience a drop in their estrogen levels, older men may have low testosterone levels (one of the risk factors for osteoporosis).

What are the risk factors for osteoporosis? There are several. First, let's look at your heredity. Did your mother and/or grandmother 'shrink' as they aged? You may have the same genes. Caucasian and Asian women tend to have lower bone density than Mediterranean, Latino or African Americans. Women with fair skin and light or red hair, or prematurely gray hair, tend to be at risk.

Small women are usually thin boned, placing them at risk. Since it seems to be fashionable to be thin as a reed, many young girls and women diet excessively. To many, this means avoiding milk and cheese because of the fat content, leading them to a low calcium diet. Anyone who has been through an eating disorder, such as anorexia or bulimia, is especially vulnerable. Fortunately, by today's standards, it is also fashionable for a woman to be athletic - not so in my day! We are making progress.

Estrogen is a great protector against bone loss. From the onset of your menstrual periods to the time they cease (menopause) your estrogen level keeps your bones strong. Postmenopausal women experience a drop in estrogen and an increased risk for bone loss. Your doctor can best advise you as to whether or not you should pursue hormone replacement therapy. Since it is so controversial, make sure you do your homework so that you can make an informed decision.

Now let's examine your lifestyle. Are you a smoker? Did you know that smoking decreases your estrogen level? If you should experience a bone fracture, it will heal more slowly than that of a non-smoker. By the time you reach eighty years of age, your bone density will be six to ten percent lower than that of a non-smoker.

Drinking too much alcohol can adversely affect your bones. According to The U.S. Department of Health and Human Services, moderate drinking (one drink per day for women or two drinks for men) may even be beneficial. If your daily consumption is more, your calcium balance could change. Consuming too much alcohol on a regular basis, could lead to a vitamin D deficiency, which in turn, can decrease your calcium absorption.

I'm sure it is no surprise that what you do, and do not eat, affects your bone health. Foods containing calcium help build and maintain strong bones. Vitamin D is necessary to aid in the absorption of calcium. Most milk purchased today is Vitamin D fortified. You can also find cereals and orange juice containing calcium and vitamin D. Sunlight is a good source of Vitamin D. All you need is ten to fifteen minutes of sun exposure, two or three times per week, to supply you with the required amount. Taking a short walk outdoors on a sunny day can do the trick. Fish and eggs also contain Vitamin D. Fruits and vegetables supply you with potassium and magnesium, helping you build calcium stores.

There is no need to panic if you are lactose intolerant. There is calcium in soymilk, and/or lactose-free milk, molasses, mineral water, nuts (almonds, pistachios, macadamias, and pecans), carrots, broccoli and spinach. Adding a calcium supplement may not be a bad idea.

Now we come to my favorite subject - exercise. The best activity to prevent or minimize Osteoporosis is weight bearing and resistance training. Weight bearing is anything that requires you to move against gravity. Walking, dancing, running, volleyball, tennis, climbing stairs, are some examples. Resistance training involves pushing or pulling and lifting. Push-ups and pull-ups, lifting free weights, and working out on weight machines all qualify as resistance training. If you are a stranger to weights and weight machines, get a professional to show you where to start. (See EXERCISE). Rubber bands, especially designed for resistance, are available in sports stores.

To keep your bones strong, you don't need to spend hours in the gym. Working out as little as forty-five minutes to an hour, twice a week, will do the trick. You can accomplish the same thing by walking briskly, for an hour, three to five times a week. The key is to experiment and find out which activity is right for you.

Now I'd like to address the parents and anyone else responsible for childcare. Everything you just read applies to young children as well as adults. The earlier they begin good nutrition and exercise, the better. Remember, they only have twenty to thirty years to build strong bones.

Teenage girls, especially those who are involved in sports such as gymnastics, figure skating, track and field and ballet, could develop Female Athletic Syndrome. Stringent dieting coupled with excessive exercise, leads to an interruption in her menstrual periods, which in turn, lowers the estrogen levels. Her bones will surely suffer from the lack of adequate nutrients and estrogen. This could lead to Osteoporosis at an early age.

Guarding against Osteoporosis is more important than ever before, simply because of the increase in life expectancy. We want those 'bonus years' to be pleasant. See you in the weight room.

PART TWO

BIRTH TO AGE SIX

ATTENTION PARENTS! If you think your pre-school children are too young to understand their surroundings, guess again. You will never again exercise more influence and control over your children than you do when they are infants to six years of age. Most psychologists agree that what children learn and experience in the formative years, stays with them for the rest of their lives, so - what better time to expose them to a healthy life style.

A prime example of children learning by exposure to their environment is the Gillespie family of Middletown, New Jersey. When Jaime Gillespie was just a toddler, Janet, her mom, often indulged in twenty-mile bike rides with baby Jaime on the back. Janet, a former competitive swimmer and avid walker, always included Jaime in all of her activities. Her husband Kerry, a seasoned competitive runner, is a strong contender in his sport. He serves on the committee that organizes and runs the annual Great Race in Middletown, New Jersey.

When Jaime was five and a half years old, the second Gillespie child, Shannon was born. Twenty-two months later, Sean arrived on the scene. The family never missed a beat. Janet was now walking three miles per day with a double stroller, while Jaime pedaled along on her bike. Every weekend Kerry was involved in running races while the whole family looked on. Meanwhile, whenever possible, Janet had all three kids in the water. The children began running with Kerry on Monday nights in the summer at Lake Takanassee. Both Kerry and Jaime have been involved in biathlons and triathlons.

When Jaime was just seven years old, she earned a place on the prestigious Red Bank YMCA Swim Team. A few years later, Shannon followed and then Sean, each one at age seven. All three children made their own decisions to do so.

Janet swims several times a week at the 'Y'. She would like to compete with the Masters Swim Team some day, but for now, she feels the children's swim meets must come first. She is content to work out in the pool several times a week and to coach the varsity swim team.

At age fourteen, Jaime emerged as an outstanding runner, cyclist and swimmer. Kerry is a distinguished runner and will no doubt continue to be for many years to come. I could go on and on about this remarkable family, but I think you get the picture.

UPDATE:

I contacted Janet recently to see if the family was still involved in sports. Where does the time go? Jaime is now 26, Shannon is 20 and Sean is 18. All three have distinguished themselves in their respective sports, earning championships and honors too numerous to mention.

Awarded a swimming scholarship to Marist College, Jaime served as captain in her senior year. After graduation, she moved to Oahu, Hawaii to teach special education for two years. While there, she participated in the Oahu 145-mile perimeter run and traveled to Japan to dance with her hula class. She is currently finishing her fourth year teaching, and will coach the Holmdel Pool Club Swim Team with her mom again this summer.

Shannon attended Red Bank Catholic High School where she excelled in cross-country, track and swimming. She earned All-American status in race walking competition in the National Junior Olympic Program. She went on to compete in running at Loyola College and set a new record in the 5K race-walk at the Penn Relays. During the summer, she competes in lifeguard tournaments for the Gateway National Park.

Sean attended Christian Brothers Academy, where he achieved top-ten honors in high school swimming, and was chosen for the All-Shore first team. He also competed at Nationals for the CBA Crew Team. Last summer, Sean was the youngest member of the Lifeguard Tournament Team for Gateway National Park. Sean will be attending the University of North Carolina at Wilmington in the fall.

Kerry is an adjunct professor for Health & Fitness at Brookdale Community College and Director of Complementary Medicine at Staten Island University Hospital. Somehow, he still finds the time and energy to compete in running and triathlon events.

Janet continues to walk, swim and cycle, in addition to her long-term positions as a swim team coach and swim instructor.

Pre-school children tend to absorb the family environment. They gravitate toward activities with which they are familiar and comfortable. In the words of Dr. Phil, "You learn what you live."

I am not suggesting that all parents must be accomplished athletes. Walking, cycling, swimming, playing ball are all things that everyone can do. Have fun with your kids. An active lifestyle, with some outdoor activity, is both healthy and fun for the whole family. Kids naturally want to do what their parents and older siblings do. It may take some effort on your part, but the benefits are well worth it.

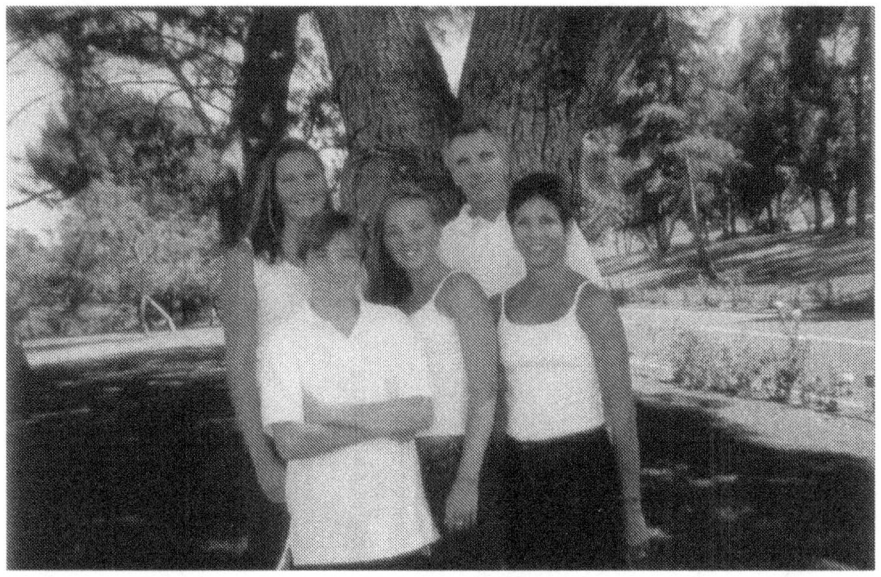

The Gillespies (2002)
(Left to right) front row - Sean, Shannon, Janet \ back row - Jamie and Kerry

Infants, toddlers, and pre-schoolers are, by nature, constantly in motion. They seem to have boundless energy. To sit them down in front of the TV, to have some peace and quiet, is tempting. Of course, they do need some down time and a little TV is fine. The four to six year olds sometimes play video games for hours. Before it becomes a major activity in their lives, you as a parent, may want to consider limiting the amount of time spent in such activities.

The YMCA offers many pre-school classes, some including a parent. The swim classes start as early as six-months old with water orientation. By the time they are three, they can take a swim class without a parent. I have had four and five year olds on my swim teams.

Good nutrition is essential at this stage of life. Breast-feeding infants, for a minimum of three months, is enormously beneficial, both nutritionally and emotionally. Mother's milk contains the nutrients the baby needs and provides immunity to several diseases. The infant is comforted and the bond between mother and child becomes established more quickly. I asked my granddaughter, who recently gave birth, shortly after she received her Registered Nurse Certification, how she coped with breast-feeding. She said that she used a combination of formula and breast-feeding; she also uses a breast pump on occasion. In her words, "Find out what works." For her, introducing formula was a good idea, since she will be working two thirteen-hour shifts a week at the hospital. While the four-month-old baby is in the care of family members, feeding will not be a problem.

At the risk of being repetitious, I will briefly mention the importance of bone health.

Specifically: building bone density. Consensus is that Osteoporosis is a pediatric disease with a geriatric outcome. An abundance of calcium is a definite need. Most young children will willingly drink milk. To guard against excess fat, you may want to give your children skim or low fat milk. If you have one of those rare kids who does not like milk, try flavoring, such as chocolate. Puddings, cheese, yogurt, and most dairy products, as well as some vegetables, contain calcium.

If your child is lactose intolerant, it is time for you to get creative – it's worth the effort. Soymilk and/or lactose-free milk, calcium-fortified orange juice, bread and cereals, molasses, mineral water, nuts (almonds, pistachios, macadamias, pecans), carrots, broccoli, spinach, are all sources of calcium. Discuss this with your pediatrician. He may suggest a calcium supplement.

Your common sense will tell you to avoid foods containing large amounts of fat and sugar. Try fresh fruit to satisfy the sweet taste most children seek. Offer your kids all foods, but do not try to force them to eat what they obviously do not like. There is no need to obsess about your children's food intake. They will eat when they are hungry. My children's pediatrician told me that most children's appetites diminish during the time they are not growing. As a mother of two daughters, I know how difficult it can be to try to get them to eat a proper diet. Do not let mealtime become battleground. Try to create a pleasant and relaxed atmosphere. Scheduling meal times works best. I am fully aware of the pressures and lack of free time parents have these days. If possible, arrange to have at least one meal per day as a family.

Have you given any thought to dental health? I realize it is not a top priority for new moms. After all, babies are born without teeth. Most parents suffer along with their children when they begin to cut teeth, somewhere around six to ten-months old. Typically, they will have all their baby teeth when they are two to two and one half.

It is not unusual for baby teeth to decay. Some dentists believe that putting a baby to bed with a bottle of milk or juice is not a good idea for healthy teeth. The sugar content in such drinks remains in the mouth all night and can lead to tooth decay. The earlier you begin cleaning those tiny teeth, the better. Most three-year olds do not yet have the coordination to use a toothbrush. You can put a little toothpaste on a cloth and wipe them off. It won't be long before they will want to do it themselves.

Four years old is a good time for your child's first dental visit. If he/she is resistant, as my daughter was, a pediatric dentist is a good choice. My daughter was a challenge, to put it kindly. Unfortunately, she had several cavities and needed extensive work. Why fill baby teeth - to maintain proper spacing for the permanent teeth.

Your little one's skin is a remarkable, multi-functioning organ. It amazes me how our skin can adapt to the growth of the body, as well as shrink with weight loss or after pregnancy. Protection for your child's 'birthday suit', especially from sun damage, is essential. You may think that only applies to summer. **Wrong!** Sun damage can occur any time the skin is exposed to its rays. Before you reach for *your* sunscreen, consider the opinion of many dermatologists who believe that a chemical-free product may be safer for your baby's tender skin. Products containing zinc oxide or titanium dioxide act as a protective barrier against sun damage and are not absorbed; an added advantage is that they are effective immediately, upon application, as opposed to those containing chemicals, which you need to apply thirty minutes before sun exposure to allow time for absorption. Your pediatrician or dermatologist is the best person to advise you on this matter.

Dermatologists believe it only takes one severe sunburn to cause permanent damage to the skin. The damage usually does not become apparent until much later in life.

Parenting is the most important job you will ever have. It is within your power to pave the way, during these formative years, to a healthy lifestyle for your child. Isn't that what you want?

SEVEN THROUGH TWELVE

Your little six-year-old people pleaser has turned seven and is displaying some assertiveness and independence. Seven-year-olds are usually in school for a full day, five days per week. Their world has expanded beyond home and family, and now they experience the ideas and attitudes of teachers, coaches and peers. The process of growing up has begun. Scary, isn't it? Brace yourself - puberty is on the way. Here is where we separate the girls from the boys.

The onset of puberty in girls usually begins at eight to ten years of age; however, it can begin as early as seven - eight and a half to eleven is the average. The physical changes include pubic hair, underarm hair and breast buds. These changes horrify some girls, while others eagerly await them. Behavioral changes, such as becoming clannish, and sometimes a tendency to be cruel, are likely. A strained relationship with the mother is common, but it's important for parents to be understanding at this time. If you realize what is going on inside them, it won't be so disturbing.

Before puberty, the average girl grows about two inches per year. During the growth spurt, they may add as much as four inches in a year. It slows down after the first menstrual period. The pelvic bones increase in size and fat deposits form, causing the hips to widen. The body becomes shapelier, and more womanly. They may add between thirty-five and fifty-five pounds before they are finished growing. That will usually happen sometime in their teens.

We are all predisposed to our body types by genetics. The three basic body types are, slim and angular, muscular with broad shoulders and slim hips, or round and softly curved. Changing this is no more possible than to change the color of our eyes. Young girls who are involved in activities, such as distance running or gymnastics and ballet, which require super-slim bodies, may not understand, nor accept, the changes in their bodies when they reach puberty. They also will not understand that they cannot choose their body type. The truth is most girls are not meant to be petite and super lean.

Trying to cling to a little girl's body can lead to the *Female Athletic Syndrome*. Low weight and long periods of training can stop menstruation, if it has started. Eating disorders are a real risk. The signs include hyperactivity, depression, moodiness, intense fear of being fat and feeling cold much of the time. In addition, yo-yo dieting can be harmful, and may result in obesity in adulthood.

My eight-year-old daughter became involved in long jumping with the town Parks Department. She was a slender child with long legs, which was ideal for the sport. She began competing and discovered that she was winning at town and county meets. It became a source of pride for her. She worked hard and continued to improve. Then disaster struck! At the age of eleven, she put on weight around the hips. She could no longer jump as high or as far, and her winning streak came to a screeching halt. She was devastated. I could see what was happening and tried to explain it to her. She hated the change in her body, and decided she was fat. Luckily, she got into another activity at which she did well, and survived the crisis.

Typically, a girl will begin to menstruate between the ages of thirteen and fourteen. Some get their first periods as young as nine or as late as fifteen. I am mentioning it in this section because your child needs to be prepared before it happens so it will not frighten her.

Boys begin puberty approximately two years after girls. The first outward sign is the growth and development of the male genitals and the beginning of pubic hair growth. Without going into detail, I will tell you that there are five stages of genital development. The first stage begins as early as nine or as late as fourteen. Stage 5 usually happens at age fourteen to sixteen. Reactions to this stage of development range from excitement to embarrassment. Boys tend to be less dramatic than girls are about these changes.

Boys grow approximately two inches per year. They add almost four inches per year during the growth spurt. It usually covers a period of three to four years and results in nine to eleven inches of added height. Most boys continue to grow at a slower rate, until they are about nineteen. Weight gain is usually included in this same growth spurt. Much of the increased weight is due to bone, internal organ and muscle growth.

Both boys and girls may add some body fat between growth spurts. There is no need for alarm. It is not an indication of future obesity. If the added fat is not lost with the next growth spurt, he/she may not be getting enough exercise or could be eating the wrong kind of food.

During this stage of life, children continue to cut permanent teeth. The side teeth come in around seven to nine years old, followed by the eyeteeth at age ten to thirteen. The twelve-year molars come in at about age eleven to thirteen. Insist, while you still can, that they brush after breakfast and dinner. Preventing tooth decay is a lifelong battle. It is never too soon to start.

Good nutrition is essential during this period of rapid growth. Again, I must mention the need for calcium in particular, during this period of bone growth. Their bones have to last a lifetime. Some foods rich in calcium include milk, cheese, yogurt, fortified cereals, orange juice, broccoli, kale, green beans and tofu. I strongly suggest that you start your child on low-fat milk now, if you haven't already done so. Hopefully, they will continue to drink milk through their teens. Their bodies no longer need the additional fat in whole milk; however, the calcium and other nutrients are essential. Thirteen-hundred milligrams of calcium per day is the suggested requirement. Most kids in this age group will willingly eat enough food, but it is up to you, as parents, to see that they eat a well-balanced diet. A daily multi-vitamin is a wise addition to the plan.

A good breakfast is necessary at this age. I know many kids will try to beg off, but stick to your guns. With all that growing going on, they cannot afford to skip any meals, especially not breakfast.

Getting plenty of exercise is essential during this period of rapid growth. I'm partial to sports. Could be, since I am an athletic trainer, I have seen the positive impact sports have on kids at this age. To illustrate, I would like to reprint one of my articles, previously published in the ***Two River Times***:

Kids in Sports

Who in these United States isn't interested in sports in one way or another? We're spectators, fans, participants, friends, and relatives of athletes. We especially like to watch our kids in their athletic endeavors as much as they enjoy our interest and pride in what they are doing.

The human animal is, by nature, competitive. I have seen this in my pre-school swim classes for three and four year olds. It startled me at first. Then I put it to a test by using it to get them to perform a skill they didn't particularly want to do. It worked! They were delighted and encouraged by their triumphs. (Anything you can do I can do better).

The competitive spirit is fun and exciting for children, but if parents and coaches do not guide them properly, it can be destructive and devastating. They must learn they can't always win and it's okay to make mistakes. They need to know that practice and hard work will help them reach their goals. As a swim team coach, I encourage them to go for a "personal best." Be lavish with praise for genuine achievement. Their confidence and enthusiasm will flourish right before your eyes.

The physical benefits derived from sports are obvious. They are gaining strength, enhancing coordination and using all their youthful energy in a positive way. But what about all the other benefits?

The next time you attend a child's sports event, notice the interaction between teammates. There's competition among them, but they root for each other and they all do their best for the team. Teammates form strong bonds, and the friendships that develop, tend to be long lasting. It's a wonderful feeling to be a contributing member in a joint effort. The first time I ever experienced it was at Senior National Olympics as I marched for New Jersey in the 'parade of the states'. I thought I'd burst with pride. No one should have to wait that long.

Most kids who are involved in sports learn to be achievers. The commitment they apply to their sports will usually spill over into other areas of their lives. They learn to manage their time efficiently. The competitive spirit, which drew them to sports in the first place, will not allow them to do anything halfway. Our swim team members demonstrate that. Most of them are honor students and usually continue on to good colleges. Scholarships for swimming are not unusual.

It never ceases to amaze me how much teachers and coaches learn from their students. It has been my unique privilege to work with some individual children from pre-school swim classes through swim team training. I have watched them develop as swimmers and blossom into confident out-going young people. They take such pride in their achievements. Motivation and self-discipline are outgrowths of the satisfaction they feel as a result of those achievements. They are surely learning a lot more than athletic skills. They are learning to play the game of life.

Last summer, the 2004 Olympic Games lured many of us to our TV sets for hours. As our budding athletes watched with awe and fascination, many of them were visualizing themselves on the field, in the pool, on the podium. Only a few will earn the privilege of representing their country in the Olympic Games, but just about everyone can represent school, town, or athletic club.

**

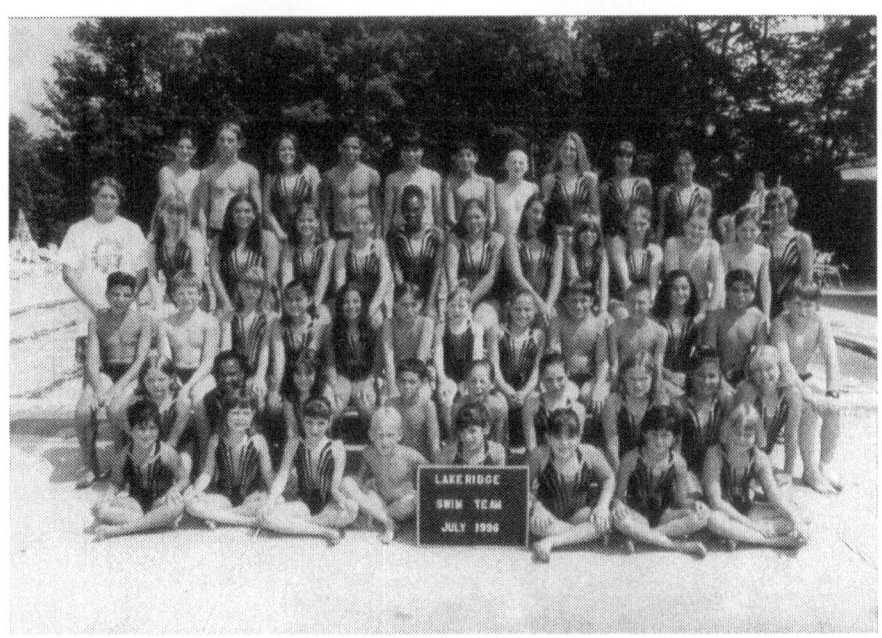

The Lakeridge Swim Team

Some children in this age group become seriously involved with their sport, particularly if they excel. We all feel pride in our accomplishments and want to continue making progress. To that end, many kids pursue weight training. In response to a question regarding weight training for a ten-year-old boy, Dr. Paul Donohue, newspaper columnist, had this to say. "Putting stress on growth plates can lead to injury. However, weightlifting doesn't stop growth unless the growth plate is disrupted by an injury. Such injuries are most uncommon. Nowadays, experts in growth, development and exercise encourage pre-pubescent children to lift weights. The relative lack of male hormone does not mean that there won't be any muscle growth. The growth just won't be as exuberant as it will be when male hormones kick in." He further states, "A parent's supervision is required to make sure the weight is not so heavy that the child cannot lift it with ease and proper form at least eight times in a row."

In today's hi-tech world, many children are spending far too much time playing video games, surfing the net and watching TV. I believe it is a major contributing factor to obesity in children. Children need physical activity and social experience with other children their own age.

The other extreme is over-scheduling our kids. Many of them have so many commitments that they are compelled to eat in the car while being transported from one activity to another. This can create pressure and poor eating habits. They need some time just to be kids.

Somewhere there is a happy medium.

THIRTEEN THROUGH EIGHTEEN

The teen years tend to be exciting, exhilarating, confusing, frightening and even depressing - or somewhere in between. The hormones are kicking in and these kids are experiencing all kinds of new feelings and emotions, not the least of which is their sexuality. Physically, they are beginning to resemble adults. To some, this means they should be treated as adults. Parents may become the enemy. After all, don't they try to stop them from doing whatever they want to do and going wherever they want to go?

A teen's physical appearance becomes important and profoundly affects his/her self-esteem. All teens want to be accepted. No one wants to be perceived as 'different'. I vividly recall the pain I experienced when my final growth spurt happened far sooner than average.

At the age of thirteen, I had reached five foot four inches and one hundred fifteen pounds. I had just begun high school and looked like a typical teenager. Pleased with my appearance, I was taken by surprise with the next phase of my growth. By the time I reached fourteen, I had grown three inches in height and gained twenty-five pounds. Now I looked like a full-grown adult and then some. My body was muscular and, to my peers, I looked just plain **big.** All I wanted to do was hide. My friend, on the other hand, two years my senior, had the opposite experience. Her body remained little girlish until she was seventeen.

For those teenagers who can relate to my experience, the good news is that the other kids will catch up within a few years. As it turned out, my growth period ended at fourteen.

Boys may have the opposite problem. While some grow and mature early, experiencing a strength spurt, due to an increase in muscle and testosterone, others remain small, thin and boyish until they are fifteen or sixteen. The early bloomers will begin to develop facial hair, a deepening voice and an Adam's apple. Those are the boys who usually excel in high school sports.

My grandson is a prime example of a male late bloomer. His appearance remained 'little boyish' until he reached sixteen. His appearance changed, it seems, overnight. He grew seven inches in one year, between sixteen and seventeen. During that rapid growth spurt, he suffered with growing pains in his back and legs.

There is virtually nothing we can do to alter the way a child develops physically, but we, as parents, can support our children and do our best to help them through this difficult stage.

It has recently been determined that the teenage brain undergoes a complete reorganization that does not end until age twenty-one or later. Could this account for the risky choices many of them make? Perhaps, perhaps not.

Parental control all but disappears when kids reach their teens. However, this is not the time to assume that, because they no longer need our help to dress and feed themselves, and they know enough not to run out into the street, they no longer need supervision.

I remember how indestructible I felt when I was a teen. I thought bad things only happened to other people. I took chances that make my hair stand on end when I recall them. As parents, watch for signs of self-destructive behavior, from drug and alcohol abuse to unprotected sex.

Teenagers tend to live in the moment. The future, to them, is something they can't imagine. All they want is to enhance their lives *now*. For me, summer was my time to shine. I knew I looked great with a tan. My skin turned golden brown, my hair bleached out and my teeth showed up beautifully white. I enjoyed much more attention from the boys. Looking back, I suspect that was due to a higher level of confidence rather than my perceived improvement in appearance. I cringe when I think of how my friends and I applied baby oil and lay in the sun for hours on end. We literally fried our skin. Many of us are paying for it now, with brown spots and skin cancer. Even though I know better now, in my teens, I think I would have done the same thing. The future doesn't seem real to kids that age.

As I mentioned before, personal appearance becomes extremely important, so when they experience any sort of disfiguration, it sends them into a tailspin. Acne is common in teens. It can seriously undermine what confidence they have built up. A dermatologist can control the skin condition, both cystic and vulgaris. I urge you to seek medical care for your teen immediately. Scarring can be prevented or, at least minimized with proper care.

As if teens don't have enough to deal with, the rate of tooth decay is at its peak. When I entered high school at the age of thirteen,

I recall being lined up with the other freshmen, outside a dental facility, awaiting a check-up. It seems that was a requirement upon entering high school. When my turn came, I was astonished to hear that I had no less than fourteen cavities. I wasn't sure I had fourteen teeth. I spent the next year getting fillings. I lost my first permanent tooth at the age of eighteen. That's far too young! Nag them, if you must, to get into the habit of brushing at least twice a day.

Many kids in this age group participate in activities such as skateboarding and contact sports. Mouth guards are recommended during these high-risk activities, to protect the teeth.

Today's teens are under more pressure than any generation before them. Most of them are college bound and need to maintain a high GPA. That's easier for some than others. Do what you can to ease the pressure. Even though they are unaware of it, they still need your support and approval.

Don't assume your teen is lazy when you can't pry him/her out of bed before noon on the weekend. Teens need ten hours sleep per night and most of them are not getting anywhere near that. They are trying to catch up. They are still growing physically and mentally.

Video games, TV and computers provide escapes from pressure for many teens. That's fine, but they also need to be physically active. Once again, I recommend sports, which also provides social interaction with other teens and coaches. Not all kids can make the cut for school sports. There are many other organizations, such as the YMCA, Girls' and Boys' clubs, athletic clubs, and privately operated swim teams, which offer team sports. The advantage of sports outside of school is that the kids can expand their social circles to include other teens they may never have met elsewhere. I joined a synchronized swim club when I was fourteen. We became a close-knit group and stayed together until we were in our early twenties. My social life revolved around that club. A co-ed group of about twenty-five or so, we literally grew up together. We always had something planned for the weekends. Besides our practices and performances, we went hiking, tobogganing, canoeing and to the beach. I don't know what I would have done socially without that club. My parents more than approved.

At every stage of life, good nutrition is important. Breakfast is a must. Make it a priority in your household for the whole family. Fast foods with high fat content should be limited. I realize you cannot control what your child eats when away from home, but do what you can.

Teenagers are my favorite age group. During my five years as the Aquatic Program Director for a busy "Y," I hired, trained and supervised about forty teenage lifeguards and swim instructors. I could not have run successful programs without them. They proved to be loyal, respectful, responsible, competent and a joy to work with. I knew I could count on them and they knew they could count on me.

The teen years can be difficult for both parents and child. They can also be fun and exciting. This is the age when most of us discover who we are and who we want to be. They are standing on the threshold of their adult lives.

NINETEEN THROUGH FORTY

Welcome to the adult world! Pretty heady feeling, right? You are now in the prime of life. How long it lasts, is up to you and your genes.

My memory of 'coming of age' is still unbelievably vivid. My parents considered me an adult when I graduated high school and had a full-time job. Not many went to college in those days, especially not the girls. There were only two professions available to women: nursing and teaching. The girls who did go to college majored in *Find a Husband 101*. The rest of us settled for jobs as waitresses, office clerks and sales clerks. My guidance counselor placed me in a defense plant as a clerk. It didn't pay well, but it was enough to cover my expenses and contribute a little to the household. My parents loosened the reigns and I began my life as a responsible adult.

In those days, clothing stores employed sales people to help customers with their selections. I finally had enough money to buy the clothing I wanted, so when the sales clerk began picking out 'slenderizing' styles for me, it forced me to face a fact I already knew; I was overweight. The minor changes I made in my daily eating habits, (see WEIGHT CONTROL/ DIET) enabled me to shed twenty pounds in two months. I certainly wasn't thin, but my athletic body was not meant to be. As far as I was concerned, I was at my *personal best.*

The following year, at age nineteen, an opportunity arose for me to pursue my dream. The synchronized swim club I mentioned in the previous section (THIRTEEN THROUGH EIGHTEEN) became the most important thing in my life. By the time we reached post-high school age, we had developed a level of skill that enabled us to perform, as a group, at many local functions. Always looking for new ideas in the sport, and for the simple pleasure of seeing a professional performance, we went to New York to see *The Aquashow.* It took place nightly, at an outdoor arena with a seating capacity of eight thousand. *The Aquashow* received reviews along with the Broadway shows. We decided that we were capable of performing as well as the swimmers in the show, so we wrote a letter to the producer. He didn't answer until the following spring. Try-outs were at an indoor pool in New York City. Four of us tried out – two did not make it. I gave it my best shot, and made the cut. It was a dream come true - getting paid for doing what I loved. There is no doubt, in my mind, that I would have missed the experience of a lifetime, had I not shed those twenty pounds. Now, I was even more determined to stay fit.

Physically, you reach maturity somewhere between nineteen and twenty-five. You are strong, flexible, and highly energetic; that is, if you are fit. To stay that way doesn't take a lot of work. If you should find yourself carrying a little extra weight, now is the time to adjust your diet and exercise to get it under control. Do not procrastinate! The longer you wait, the harder it will become. The usual healthy diet, moderate exercise and good posture should do it. It will take many more years of life's experiences to mature mentally, emotionally and spiritually.

Many of you will begin some sort of higher education; and that may mean living away from home and fending for yourself for the first time in your young life. Choices made now can and will profoundly affect your future. Experimenting with drugs, alcohol and unprotected sex may seem like fun to you right now; however, the consequences of such choices are not. No lecture, I promise. I'm sure you won't have to look far to see the results of someone's single unwise choice. Party hearty, my young friends, but ***please***, use your common sense. Your life depends on it. Enough said - you get the picture.

Once you reach physical maturity, you may begin to settle into habits that you won't even notice; specifically, the way you stand, sit and walk. Slumping the shoulders, which many of us do, especially when we are tired, can lead to the beginning of muscle imbalance in the shoulder area. Here is how it happens. The body adapts itself to our habits, consequently, the muscles at the front of the shoulders shrink and the opposing muscles stretch, making it difficult to straighten up. Proper body alignment is easier to maintain than to fix. Poor posture can also cause protrusion of the abdomen and crowding of the internal organs. Your lungs may have difficulty expanding to their full capacity.

Sitting hunched over a desk all day causes fatigue in the neck, shoulders and lower back. It's a good idea to stretch the shoulders and neck a couple of times during the workday. Pinch the shoulders together, then roll them forward and back. To stretch your neck, look over your shoulder on each side, and hold for about ten seconds.

Stretch your ear to your shoulder on each side, again holding for ten seconds. It's okay to do neck rolls, but only from shoulder to shoulder, never back.

Getting into the habit of proper body alignment (good posture) at this age, can save you a lot of unnecessary back pain. A good recliner, which supports your back and head, as well as your legs, can allow you to relax, while at home, without compromising your posture. My mom always said, "Try the chair to see if it fits you." That is not as crazy as it sounds. We come in all sizes, and the chair you select needs to have the proper contours for *you*.

As we approach thirty, subtle physical changes begin to occur. The first visible sign is in the skin. There is a physiologic slowdown of the cellular system. Skin texture becomes coarser. Your inherent tendencies toward facial expressions: the way you smile, knit your brow, and squint, begin to surface, particularly around the mouth. If you are genetically predisposed, hair will begin to thin, especially in men.

Early to mid-thirties, is a good time to check for oiliness in your skin. It may be changing. As a teenager, I battled the effects of oily skin and hair. It never occurred to me that this condition could change. It wasn't until I went to a cosmetic shop with a friend that I discovered my skin had changed. When the cosmetologist told me that my skin was dry, I did not believe her. I thought she just wanted to make a sale. A closer look and touch convinced me she was right. Moisturizers are essential for both face and body. At the very least, they minimize both the look and feel of dry skin. Don't forget to protect your skin from sun exposure, even in winter.

In the late thirties, the inner lining of the skin begins to lose fat, causing a change in the contours of the face. If the change bothers you, there are many treatments available to minimize the effects of this natural process.

As I mentioned previously, **(see Weight Training)** both men and women begin losing strength, muscle and bone mass after thirty. This is the time to get serious about keeping in shape. To slow down the natural progression of bone loss, weight-bearing exercise is necessary. Aside from working out with weights, anything with impact or resistance will do the trick. Walking, jogging, playing basketball, softball, volleyball, or any activity involving impact will work. Resistance exercises, such as push-ups and rubber band stretching also qualify. Thirty minutes, three times per week, should be enough for bone health. Of course, you will need calorie burning and flexibility exercises as well, to maintain your fitness.

You are now at the stage of life when you may be taking on the responsibilities of career, family, or both. Falling into unhealthy lifestyle habits becomes easy and comfortable. Your time becomes limited. Eating on the run, not getting enough sleep, and not taking time out for yourself and your needs, often becomes a way of life. It does not have to be that way.

We are equipped today with the knowledge we need to slow the aging process. I'm hearing and reading that, "Today's fifty is yesterday's thirty." The most obvious example I can think of, is the longevity of a professional athlete's career, as compared to a generation ago. In addition, amateur athletes are so numerous, that competitive Masters Programs are growing in almost every sport. Senior Games (competitive sports for people fifty and over) are growing in both numbers of athletes and sports choices. Once again, I would like to mention that my Masters teammates, at ages thirty-four and fifty, both completed the swim across the English Channel, and are now in the record books.

Rumor has it that our metabolism begins to slow down in the thirties and forties. Maybe so, but I can't say that I noticed it. As I mentioned earlier, (see **Weight Control**) we have some control over our own metabolism. In my opinion, we slow down, not our metabolism. My daughter, who is educated on the subject, disagrees with me. Her opinion is that I compensated for the change by adjusting my diet and exercise. She may be correct. I always kept a close eye on my weight and cut calories if the weight gain reached five pounds. If you agree with my daughter, do not let it be an excuse for gaining weight. Now is when you may have to make a choice. It's up to you.

Sometime in my mid to late thirties, my kids were in school full time and I found I had more time to myself. Once they were off to school, I started to crawl back into bed, snuggle under the covers and turn on the TV. Sometimes, I'd stay there until about ten o'clock. Although I enjoyed the luxury, a red flag flashed in my head. This could become a habit. I felt guilty and the word 'lazy' crept into my head. That is when I decided to get a part-time job, which enabled me to be there for the kids when they came home from school and still have time to look after the household chores and cook for my family. I put my earnings into a savings account and later used it to finance both my daughters' weddings.

Approaching forty is panicsville for many of you. It shouldn't be. By that time in your life, your career is probably established and the kids are well on their way. If you have been living a fit and healthy lifestyle, you should have many more years to look and feel your best. Personally, I believe I looked my best between the ages of thirty and fifty. At thirty, I was married and a stay-at-home mom with two daughters. By that time, I was mature and confident enough to develop my own style. Staying fit was always a priority for me. It allowed me to enjoy every stage of life to its fullest.

I celebrated my fortieth birthday by redecorating my home and inviting all of my friends to my birthday party. With my children almost grown, I had a little more freedom to pursue more of my own interests. My girls and I took jazz lessons together and practiced in the family room. Keeping up with them was not a problem. I only stopped going when the teacher kept insisting that I perform in the recital. That's where I drew the line.

The forties is a fun time. So what if you see a few lines and wrinkles appearing? Obsessing over lost youth can prevent you from enjoying your present life. As long as you are fit, trim, look your best, and take care of your skin, you will be ***Your Personal Best***.

THE CHILDBEARING YEARS

For most women, early adulthood once meant the beginning of the childbearing years. Biologically, a woman can become pregnant from the beginning of her menstrual cycle up to menopause. Because of the many remarkable changes taking place in today's high-tech world, the childbearing years are no longer restricted to a specific age group. Many women are choosing to concentrate on their careers, and postpone starting a family until their forties. Single women are opting to become mothers. Grandmothers are even bearing their own grandchildren! Now there's one for the books! Just a few short years ago, these things were not even considered viable options.

This is a complete reversal of what was previously considered 'the natural order of life'.

These are not your mother's childbearing years!

Time was, when a woman began bearing children, it was a given that she would lose her figure and begin to look matronly. We now know better. Once fitness came to the forefront of our awareness, young mothers realized that they had control over what happens to their bodies after giving birth. Of course, the better your fitness level before you become pregnant, the easier it will be to get back into shape after the baby is born.

Seek pre-natal care the minute you suspect you are pregnant. Your health care professional will advise you how to best care for yourself and your baby. He/she will guide you through your nutritional needs, weight gain and restrictions on exercise. I believe that you can continue most activities that you have been doing. This is not the time in your life to start something new or try to lose weight.

Regular exercise for a minimum of thirty to forty-five minutes, three to five times a week, is necessary to maintain your fitness level. Avoid high intensity aerobics, jerky or bouncy movements, deep flexion or extension of joints, jumping, jarring motions or rapid changes in direction. Overheating can harm both you and your baby. Your body's 'air-conditioning' system is less efficient during pregnancy. For that reason, avoid the use of a hot tub or sauna.

Walking and/or swimming are my first recommendations. Both activities are safe and comfortable for your changing weight and center of gravity. I also recommend water exercise (surprise, surprise) as long as the water is not more than eighty-five degrees. As your pregnancy progresses and you become heavier, the buoyancy of the water allows you to move in relative comfort. Stretching in water is easier than on land. Your stretches should be mild at this time. Whatever your choice of exercise, always include a warm-up, aerobic section, strength and flexibility, and warm-down.

The female body is designed to bear children. Your body will go through many hormonal and physiological changes when you become pregnant. You may experience some emotional effects, due to the hormonal upheaval. It is not unusual to have periods of crying over what you consider nothing. Don't be alarmed. This too shall pass.

The uterus increases in size, strength and thickness as the pregnancy progresses. Your breasts will increase in size and weight. As the fetus grows and your weight increases, your center of gravity will change. This can put a strain on your back. Maintaining good posture will help. You will have an increase in blood supply of about 25% to 50%. Your heart may beat a little faster.

As your abdomen begins is expand, you may notice the appearance of stretch marks and, perhaps, some itching. The application of lotions containing cocoa butter may help both conditions. Don't forget your breasts. They are also expanding.

By using sunscreen, and wearing a hat or visor when you are outdoors, you can protect yourself from pregnancy mask, (chloasma or melasma). It is an excess of pigmentation on the upper lips, cheeks and forehead. It may develop during pregnancy due to elevated hormone levels.

Hormonal changes may cause morning sickness. It usually occurs during the first three months. If you are lucky, you may escape it altogether. I experienced it during my first pregnancy but not the second.

To minimize your discomfort, you can do several things:

- Sit on the side of the bed for a few minutes after you wake up in the morning.
- Avoid having an empty stomach by eating five or six small meals each day.
- Eat dry toast, crackers, a peeled apple or a plain potato.

- Avoid drinking citrus juice, water, milk, coffee and tea first thing in the morning.
- Avoid any smells that nauseate you.

During your pregnancy, it is best to avoid artificial sweeteners, alcohol, smoking, caffeine, salt and processed food. You will need calcium rich food, protein, bread, cereals and fruits and vegetables. This may not be easy while you are experiencing morning sickness. I remember not being able to tolerate anything other than milk shakes and pizza.

Your health care professional will probably prescribe vitamin supplements. My doctor once told me, "Your baby will take what it needs. If you do not get enough nutrients, you will be left deficient." He also recommended that I visit the dentist. I am glad I followed his advice - I had developed several cavities.

Your baby has finally arrived! You look at this perfect miniature person you created (all by yourself) and your pride and joy overwhelms you. You have waited a long time for this moment. From here on, your doctor is the only person to guide you through postpartum and the special needs you may have following delivery, such as preparing you for breast-feeding, when you should resume exercising and dietary needs.

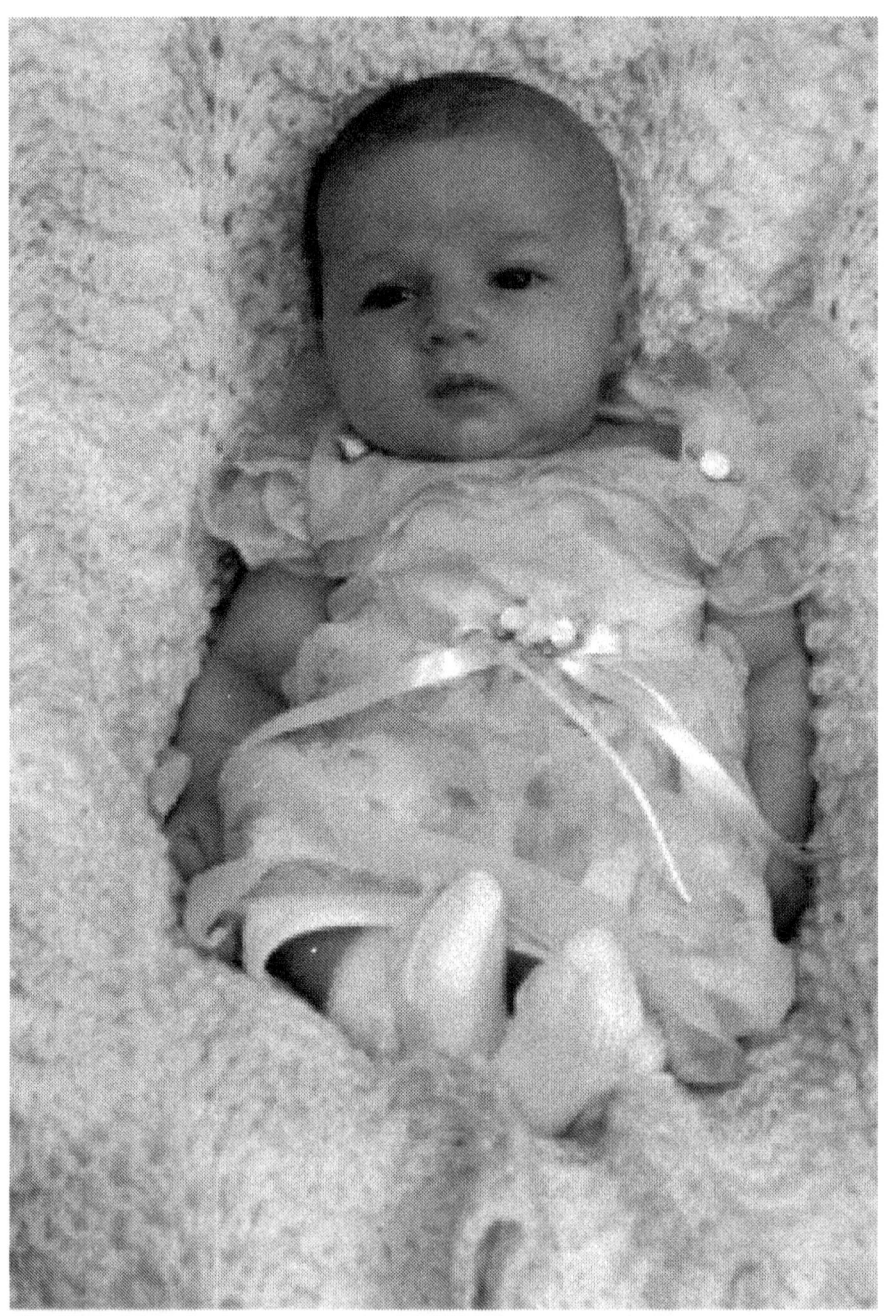

Makayla Kondreck, Author's great-granddaughter.

FORTY-ONE THROUGH SIXTY

You have reached the stage of life most of us label the 'middle years'. We conjure up an image of 'middle-age-spread' - pure Edith and Archie Bunker. Men expect to develop a paunch, while women see themselves as thickening around the middle. Inevitable? **No way!**

Recently, a magazine I have never heard of showed up in my mailbox. After I recovered from the shock of the publication name, *Geezer Jock*, I leafed through the pages to see what it was all about. Being a life-long swimmer, I went straight to the profile of a swimmer, bearing a photo of a sixty-year-old man, with a shock of gray hair and a typical perfectly toned swimmer's body. Even I was stunned to read that his fifty-meter freestyle (25.54 seconds) was a full second faster than Olympic gold medalist Jeff Farrell's record set in 1960. Then I looked at his training regimen (seven days a week). It would be an ambitious schedule for a nineteen-year-old.

The magazine went on to profile *Geezer Jock* of the year, fifty-four-year-old, Bill Collins, who looked extremely fit. A woman in her fifties, after diving competitively for only seven years, won three gold medals in the World Master's Games and continues to win in National games. Let's not forget the fifty-year-old female, who completed the swim across the English Channel in 2004, in record time.

Granted, these are the exceptions, not the rule. Most of us are not world-class athletes. However, equipped with today's knowledge, we know that physical deterioration does not occur at this age, unless we allow it. This is not the time of life to give up and let it happen. Is maintaining your fitness worth a little effort? It's your choice.

Although it is true that our capacity for fitness begins to diminish at age thirty at approximately one percent per year, (see Aging) it does not mean you have no control. Now is the time to take stock of where you are on the fitness scale.

Consider this: according to the latest life-expectancy tables, if you are forty-years old, all of your body parts need to last for at least another forty years. The only way that's going to happen, is if you make an effort now, to keep your bones, muscles, joints, heart and lungs in working order. You probably can't imagine yourself as a senior citizen at this stage of your life, nor do you want to. Okay! I get that. But, what about the here and now? Don't you want to look and feel your best?

I hear many people in this age group complain of low energy. They say they are too tired after a long day's work to exercise. Want more energy? Try a good workout. You may be surprised to discover how energized you'll feel afterwards.

Carrying around extra weight can drain you. If you have fallen victim to creeping weight gain, (see Diet and Weight Control) you need to deal with it **now**! Obesity has become a major health problem in the United States. As you already know, it can lead to other health problems and directly cause premature aging diseases such as diabetes and joint deterioration. Cutting calories is not the whole answer. Exercise is a major part of weight control. You're still young enough to handle a fairly high intensity work-out, as long as you start out slowly and work up to it. If you are totally out of condition, you may need some professional guidance. Consult your doctor before you embark on an ambitious fitness regime.

Your exercise program should encompass weight-bearing exercise for bone strength, aerobics for heart and lungs, strength training and stretching for flexibility (see Exercise).

From now on, maintaining your fitness level will keep you looking and feeling younger than your chronological age. Let's not use 'middle-age' as an excuse.

Having a mid-life crisis? Why not try something new? Nothing will revitalize you like a new venture or activity. Try something that you and your significant other can both enjoy. If you are without a significant other, your range of choices widens. My husband and I took up ballroom dancing in our forties and had the time of our lives. We went to the studio three nights a week and frequented the ballrooms in New York City on the weekends. It was fun to show off our new dancing skills at social events.

Speaking of trying something new, about a month ago, after noticing a few of my water exercise students showed some fear in the water, I asked them if they would be interested in a learn-to-swim class. To my surprise, they accepted with enthusiasm. By the second lesson, they were all maneuvering in the water without help. I'm happy to say, they are so excited and proud to be able to overcome their fear and are striving to improve their newfound skills. What is more amazing is they are in their late fifties and early sixties.

When I reached sixty, I was lucky enough to find a new career. It happened quite by accident. After relocating to a different part of the state, I could not find a job as a bookkeeper, despite an impressive resume. In desperation, I went to the local YMCA seeking a part-time job teaching swimming. Within two months, they offered me the job of Aquatic Director. It changed my life! I looked forward to going to work every day. There was always something new to learn and new challenges to meet. I am grateful every day of my life that someone gave me the chance to do a job I loved, despite my age.

You are not old until you think you are. Staying active and fit will lift your spirits and make you more fun to be with. This is a wonderful time of life. Enjoy it!

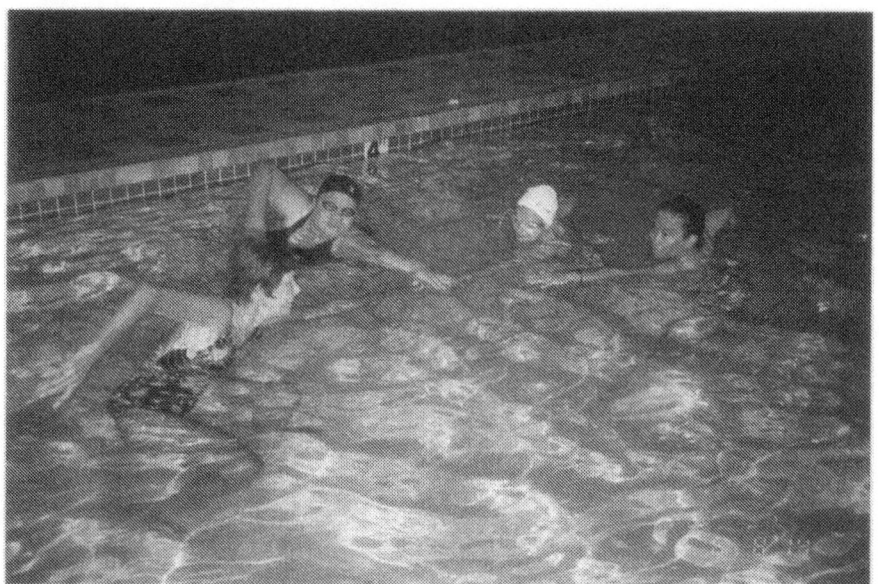

The author teaches a learn-to-swim class.

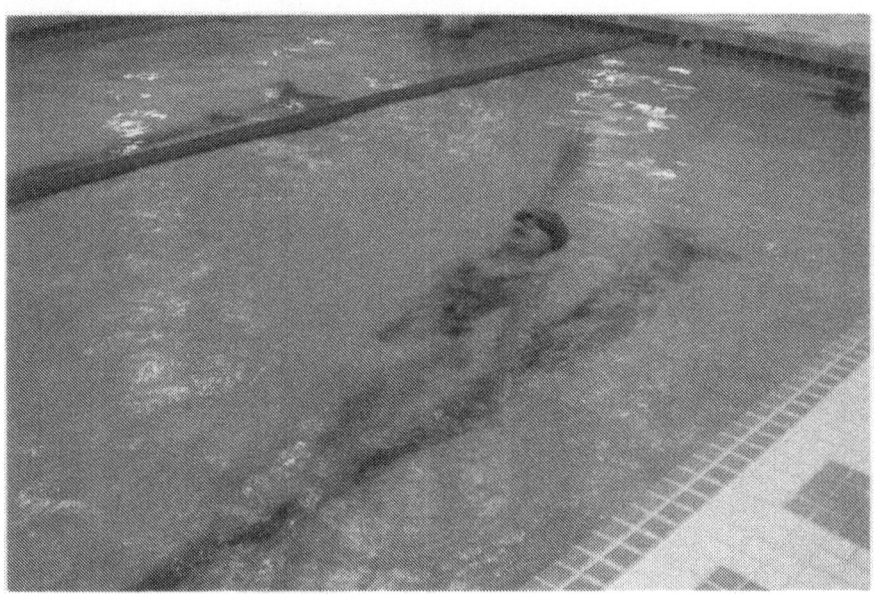

Fifty-year old Helen Lam went from non-swimmer to fitness-
swimmer in four months.

MENOPAUSE

What is it? Webster's Dictionary defines it as "the permanent cessation of menstruation." It can only be determined after you have been free of menstrual bleeding for a full year. Generally, your genes pre-determine when you begin to menstruate and when you stop. The average age is between fifty and fifty-one; however, it can occur as early as thirty or as late as fifty-eight. What precedes menopause (pre-menopause) is what most of us think of as 'the change of life'. This transitional period can take anywhere from ten to fifteen years. Herein lies the culprit.

During this time, your ovaries gradually stop producing eggs and a large amount of hormones. Emotional, intellectual and physical changes take place. You may experience irregular periods, hot flashes and vaginal dryness. Heavy bleeding may be normal at this time, but have it checked out if it persists. Not only could it be a symptom of something more serious, there is also a risk of developing anemia.

After menopause, your body produces less estrogen than before. The amount of adrenal estrogen varies greatly. You can help your adrenal glands produce a healthful supply after menopause by exercising and maintaining some body fat (not too much). A little body fat means not below fifteen percent but not over twenty-five percent. Your diet should include plenty of nutrients, especially vitamins B and C. Avoid excessive amounts of coffee, alcohol and sugar. 'Change of life' is the butt of many jokes. If you are one who is experiencing severe symptoms, it is anything but funny. When I was a teenager, I recall seeing my mom's glasses actually fog up during a hot flash. Such obvious signs of hot flashes can be embarrassing.

Some of us suffer varying degrees of symptoms. I didn't have hot flashes in the daytime, but at night, I was often awakened by night sweats so severe that I was saturated with perspiration and needed a complete change of night clothing. That lasted long after menopause. I am grateful that I got through the process without too much discomfort.

You, who are having a difficult time, may seek hormone replacement therapy. Before you do, educate yourself about the risks and benefits, then discuss them with your doctor. Hormone replacement therapy can relieve hot flashes and night sweats, relieve vaginal dryness and reduce bone loss. It will not, however, relieve depression, prevent wrinkles or prevent weight gain. Changes in your skin will become obvious. Menopause is not the culprit. It is the aging process. Your skin has two main layers: the thin outer epidermis and the thicker underlying dermis. The epidermis constantly regenerates itself.

The dermis makes up eighty-five percent of the skin's thickness. It contains nerve endings, blood vessels, sweat glands, oil glands and hair follicles. Collagen and elastin fibers make up the bulk of the dermis. As we age, the collagen and elastin begin to deteriorate. Skin loses its elasticity. The dermis becomes thinner and less efficient in retaining water. Less body fat is stored under facial skin. Sweat and oil glands slow down, producing less moisture and resulting in gradual drying, wrinkling and sagging skin.

To relieve itchiness and discomfort caused by dry skin, avoid frequent showering and bathing. Moisturizing soap is helpful, but use sparingly. Use a moisturizer after bathing while the skin is still damp. It works by creating a seal over the skin to keep water from evaporating from the top layer of the skin.

Bone loss speeds up for the first three to seven years after menopause and then slows down. The older we get, the less efficient our bodies become at absorbing calcium from food. There are many factors leading up to osteoporosis after menopause. Among them are early menopause (before forty-five), family history, amount of calcium in the diet, drop in estrogen level, small bone structure, no pregnancies, low body weight, smoking, too much caffeine or alcohol, lack or exercise and some medications.

Menopause is a transitional stage of life for women. It marks the end of the childbearing years and the beginning of new freedoms. Just think - no more painful menstrual periods and no more worries about becoming pregnant! For most of you, your child-rearing years are over and you can look forward to spending your spare time pursuing activities for which you never had the time. The best advice I can give you now, is to get on a wellness program that includes weight bearing and aerobic exercise. Make sure to have annual medical check-ups and the prescribed preventative testing. You owe it to yourself and your family to stay healthy and fit.

SIXTY-ONE THROUGH SEVENTY-FIVE

As you approach your sixties and seventies, you may experience the onset of one or more chronic and/or degenerative diseases (See Aging). The most common of these is osteoarthritis. It can range from a slight nuisance to outright disability. Joint replacement, essentially hip and knee, are common (see Arthritis). Your skin becomes thinner and drier. You may notice some gum recession. That's the bad news. The good news is that most of these conditions are manageable. It is up to you. Good health care at this stage of life is essential.

To protect your thinning skin, avoid prolonged time in a hot tub, bath or shower. Use sun block, or at least sun screen each time you experience exposure to the sun. Use a body moisturizer daily, especially after bathing. I developed winter eczema from being in a warm pool for extended periods. I was convinced the chemicals caused it. The dermatologist assured me it was a result of my aging skin's exposure to warm water for long periods. He advised limiting my time in the warm pool and applying moisturizer after my shower - while my skin was still damp. It worked.

As for your dental health, regular check-ups and cleaning can avoid loss of teeth due to gum disease. Treatment of gum recession and bone disease may be relatively easy if caught early. If not, you could lose teeth or be subjected to bone surgery.

Retaining your teeth is not the only reason to maintain proper dental health. Gum disease and the bacteria in plaque can increase your risk of more serious diseases, such as heart disease and stroke. Plaque, a thin film of bacteria, is constantly building up on the teeth and, if not removed daily, the bacteria can find its way into your bloodstream, contributing to clogged arteries and damaged heart valves.

Now that you know how important good dental health is to your overall health, you won't mind taking a little extra time to maintain good dental hygiene. To keep the bacteria to minimum, daily flossing and brushing twice a day should do the trick. Add an annual or semi-annual cleaning and you will have done your part.

Once I reached my sixties, I thought it would be down hill from then on, no matter what I did. I'm happy to say I was wrong! What I'm about to share with you, I did not learn from a book. I decided to compete in Senior Games, at the state level, when I was sixty-two. I was never a competitive swimmer and this was my first try. Much to my surprise, I qualified for nationals. As the Aquatic Director at the YMCA, I had access to a few swim team coaches. When I asked them to help me train for nationals, they readily agreed. It became a community project at the "Y." They would make sure I had all the knowledge and skills I needed to be at the top of my game. I had approximately a year to get into competitive swimming shape. I signed up for the national meet. As I was beginning to train, I had my body composition measured. (Percentage of fat vs. lean body mass). About two months into my training regimen, several people began commenting on the muscle definition beginning to appear on my back. Of course, I never look at my back, so I didn't notice the change. I was sixty-two. I couldn't possibly be building muscles at this age, could I? I did notice the increased aerobic endurance and strength in my whole body. By the time I got to nationals, I was ready.

The nationals were at Syracuse University. There were about eight thousand senior athletes looking forward to competing in their favorite sport. Ranging in age from sixty to ninety-nine, they demonstrated high levels of energy and, more importantly, a zest for life. I was more than impressed. In my early sixties, I was one of the kids. Watching people in their eighties and nineties practice and compete with enthusiasm and skill in their sports astonished me. A few had physical disabilities, but that did not slow them down. Everyone was having a great time. The most important thing, for most of us, was not winning a medal. We all qualified at the state level and were here to experience national competition. For me, meeting and interacting with athletes from all over the United States, was the most enjoyable experience. I was proud to be one of them. I came away with a sense of what a positive outlook can do for seniors. Even though they were in the twilight years of their lives, they strived to make tomorrow better than today. **That** is the attitude that keeps us young, active and living for what today and tomorrow may bring. Now that I am a senior, I consider each day a gift that I do not want to waste.

I visited the health fair while I was there. Among the tests offered, was a body composition make-up, like the one I had before

I began training. Although I only lost five pounds during my year of training, I found that I had gained five pounds in lean body mass (bone and muscle) and lost ten pounds in body fat, bringing my percentage of body fat down to eighteen percent, which is the low end of normal for a female my age. That experience taught me that it is possible to improve your fitness level considerably after sixty. Now I was convinced never to allow myself to become unfit.

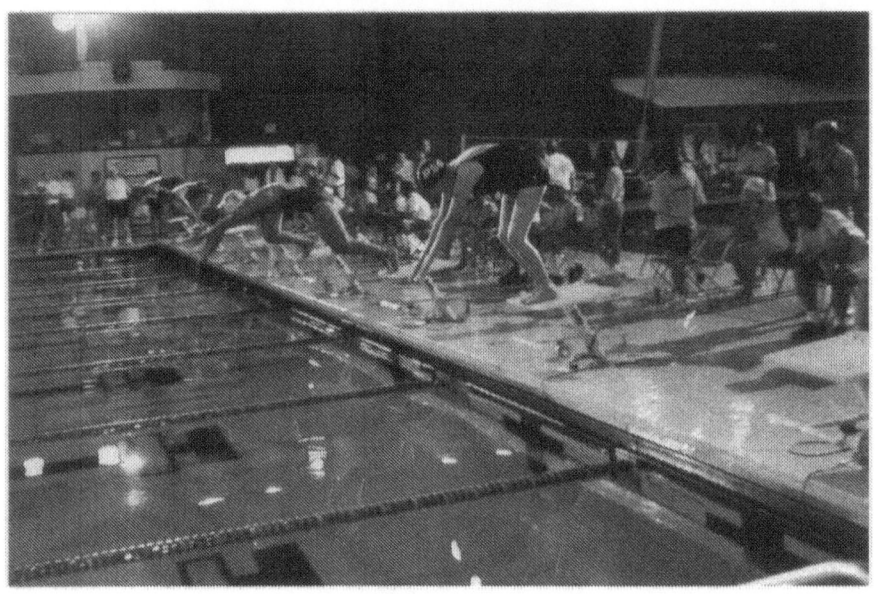

The author (second from right) competing in National Senior Olympics.

This stage of life may be a good time to re-invent ones self. Don't allow your life to become boring. This generation of seniors has more opportunities for activities than ever before. Senior centers and health clubs are offering things like art, dance, bridge, fitness classes and so much more. Try something new or volunteer to teach something in which you may excel.

You may experience some major changes in your life. Chronic health problems may force you to put some restrictions on your present life style. In addition, people nowadays are more mobile than any generation preceding us. Very few of us remain in the same place we were born. Jobs and economic conditions may take us to different parts of the country. That can cause separation anxiety. The loss of a spouse, or separation from your children and grandchildren, is difficult, to say the least. You also may find yourself living alone after sharing your residence with family. Occasionally we need to look inside ourselves and get our bearings. Staying physically and socially active can help you through such trying times. Two years ago, I relocated clear across the country. I confess, I went through about a year of separation anxiety. It took a conscious effort to get through it. I have always found that finding a way to give to others helped me. In addition, it helps to treat every day as the first day of the rest of your life. Many seniors tend to live in the past. Remember the 'good old days' but live today.

A wellness program at this stage of life is essential. Some Medicare supplemental insurance plans include a membership to a health club. The medical profession is now beginning to realize the importance of physical activity for seniors. We have come a long way in our knowledge of fitness for seniors. In my parents' generation, people over sixty, dressed and behaved like elderly people.

In order to have the ability to perform everyday activities, such as cleaning the house, doing yard work and shopping, we must maintain our strength and flexibility. Our independence depends on it. Resistance training and plenty of stretching exercises, along with twenty to thirty minutes of aerobics, will enable you to stay fit. If you have some physical restrictions, you can still get the exercise you need. Water exercise is especially beneficial for this age group.

I am currently a water-fitness professional, for the newest, largest and most well equipped athletic club in all of Las Vegas. This is the third time I have come out of retirement. I thought that not working would be easy, but I guess I'm not ready for that yet. I am happy to say that we have a large percentage of seniors, working at staying fit. I teach Arthritis classes, Ai Chi, and water jogging, a high intensity aerobics class. My students are moms, expectant moms, grandmothers, grandfathers and everyone in between. Their fitness levels are as varied as they are.

Since this section is about the sixty-one through seventy-five age group, I would like to mention one student in particular. The day that sixty-four-year-old Grace joined my water jogging class, I couldn't help but notice her. She not only looked fit and trim, she was highly energetic. Once in the water, she set the pace for those around her. I assumed she was a runner, swimmer, tennis player or some kind of athlete involved in a fast-paced sport. After class, I asked her what she does to stay so fit. She replied, "I have been doing water aerobics for ten years and find, for me, it is the best form of exercise since no pressure is put on the joints. It is also a great way to meet new people with whom you already have something in common. It's just a lot of fun especially when you have a great teacher! I believe with exercise, a good diet, lots of laughing and everything in moderation, that life can be good and hopefully long." When I asked her what she does for fun, she told me that she and her husband go camping in their motor home, go kayaking, walking, play tennis, bike ride, play all water sports and ski a little. They are planning to take up golf in the near future. Now I know why she is always smiling. She is a prime example of the healthy, active senior, enjoying life to the fullest.

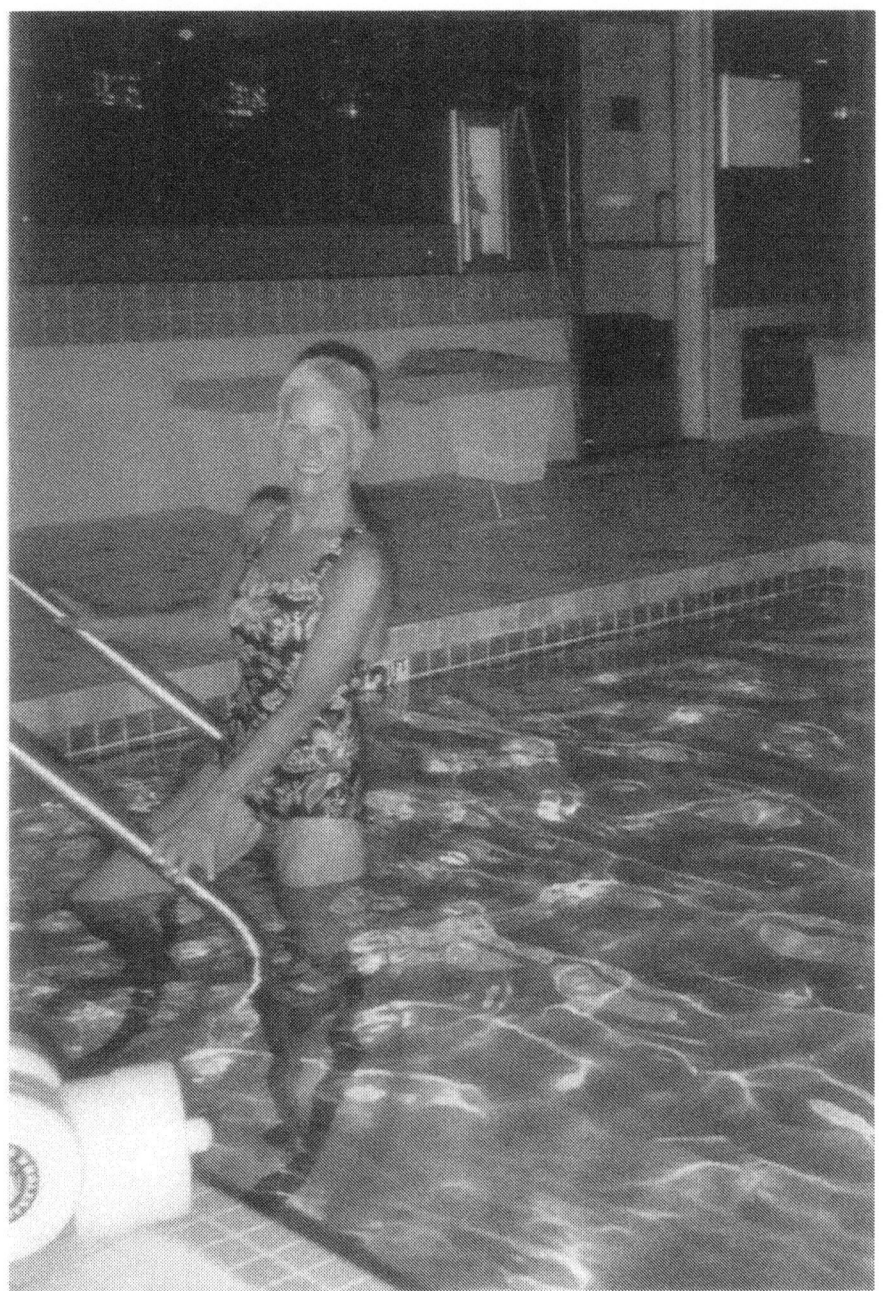

Grace Alvarez exiting the pool after class.

I am partial to water exercise for seniors for the following reasons:

- Minimal impact is less stressful on the joints.
- Stretching while in water is safer than on land.
- People with balance problems are less likely to fall.
- Water offers resistance to develop strength and aerobic fitness.
- People who have difficulty walking can still maneuver in water.
- Many exercises performed suspended in water create no impact at all.

While I was training for competition, between the ages of sixty-two and seventy-five, I was in the best physical condition of my life. I found that remarkable, for someone who was fit to begin with. Weight training, which I had never done before, was part of my training regimen. I never felt better and, I might add, have never been happier.

Just a word of caution - if you have been inactive, or only mildly active, up to this point, ease into an exercise program slowly, and gradually add length of time spent and intensity. Walking is a great way to start.

Try to get a good night's sleep and rest frequently during the day. An afternoon nap is something I indulge in on a regular basis.

These can be wonderful years. Get out and have fun!

SEVENTY-SIX AND OVER

Are you over seventy-five? Now you're in my league. As I put pen to paper, I am seventy-eight. I have come out of retirement, for the third time, to teach water exercise; and it is the joy of my life. I'm happy to say that I have many students in our age group. One woman in my Arthritis class proudly announced that she is eighty-eight. She deserves to be proud of herself. Her posture is erect and she has freedom of movement - that is no accident of fate. She has obviously worked at it.

At this stage of life, you are still responsible for your fitness. I know, many of you have physical restrictions and chronic illnesses. You may not feel much like moving around. However, as your physician will tell you, daily exercise is essential. Lack of movement will bring on quick deterioration of the muscles. In order to remain physically independent, you must be strong enough to perform the tasks of everyday living. Shopping, climbing stairs, cooking, cleaning and lifting, all require strength, especially in the legs. As mentioned previously, your legs begin losing strength in your mid-thirties. It is up to you, as individuals, to keep your legs functional. Anyone who has had a hip or knee replacement and has undergone physical therapy afterwards, knows what it takes to restore muscle strength. This morning, one of my students asked me for leg strengthening exercises. She said she could no longer get up onto the riser to sing in the choir. That may not sound like a serious problem, but to her, it is important.

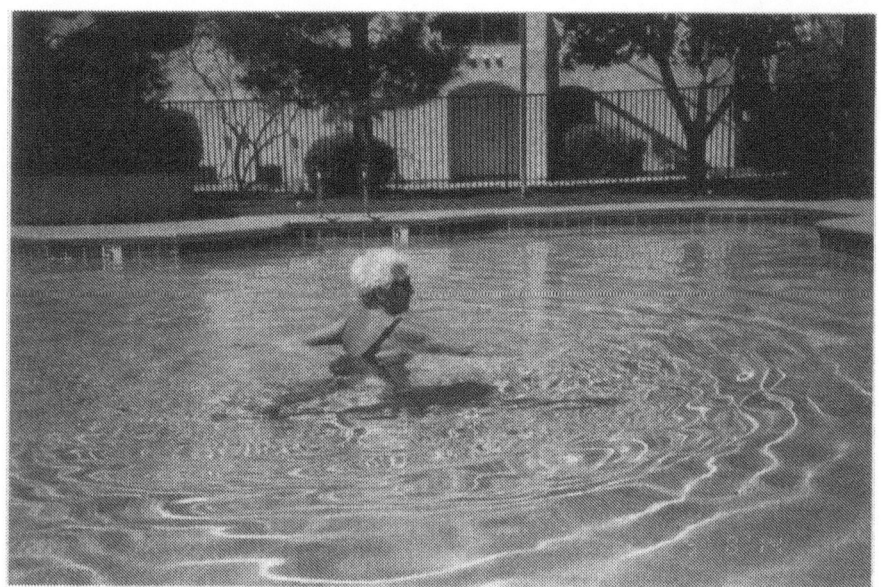

Seventy-six year old Alice Faul power walking in the pool at her condo complex.

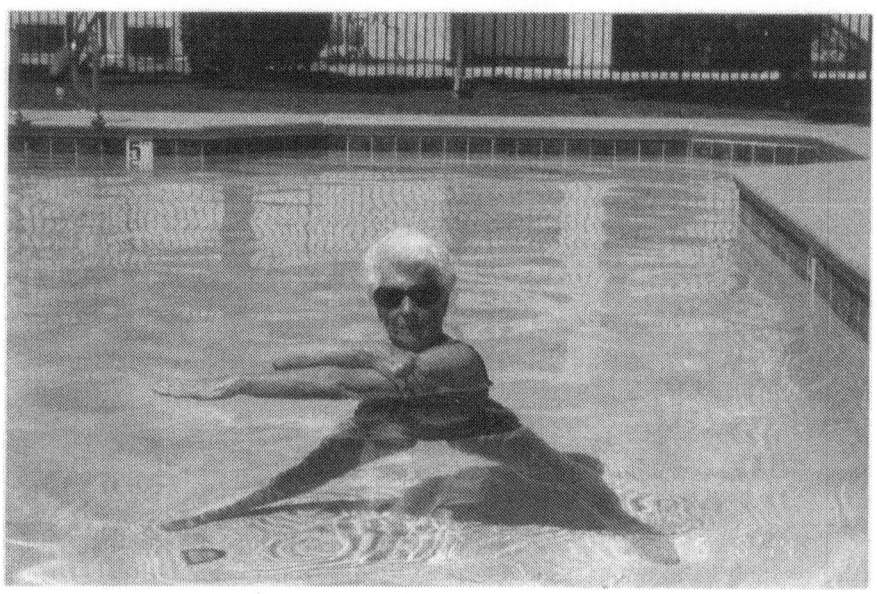

Alice stretches after her thirty-minute workout.

If you have not already done so, please read the previous section (SIXTY-ONE THROUGH SEVENTY-FIVE). Most of that applies to you.

As we age, our senses undergo some changes. Our hearing, sight, sense of taste and smell, are likely to become less sharp. Many of these changes are medically treatable.

HEARING:

Thirty to eighty percent of American adults over sixty-five have some hearing loss. Constant exposure to loud noises, even more than aging, can contribute to this condition. It happens so gradually that you may not notice until the sounds you are hearing (such as TV) seem muffled and difficult to understand. You may hear ringing or ear noises. If you have any of the above symptoms, visit an audiologist for evaluation and treatment. There are several devices available to help you hear more clearly. In addition, you can ask others to speak directly to you so that you can both see and hear them. When you attend meetings, lectures or other functions, seek out the location of a loudspeaker and sit near it. Above all, do not allow yourself to become isolated because you cannot hear everything clearly.

SIGHT:

We are now at the age when we are vulnerable to eye diseases, such as, cataracts, glaucoma, macular degeneration and cornea disease. We can also be affected by excessive tearing and dry eyes. There are medical treatments and procedures for all of the above.

Cataracts are the most common of all eye problems for seniors. The surgical procedure involves removing the clouded lens and replacing it with a permanent artificial one. I have had both my eyes done and now only need glasses for reading. My ninety-year-old friend said she has her teenage eyes again. The operation, usually performed on an outpatient basis, is quick and painless. The recuperation time is only a few days.

Glaucoma is easily diagnosed by measuring the pressure inside the eye. It is usually part of a routine eye examination. Left untreated, it can cause damage to the optic nerve and potential loss of vision. The regular use of prescription eye drops is a highly successful treatment.

The symptoms for macular degeneration include distorted vision, seeing dark spots, and diminishing clear color vision. If diagnosed in the early stages, laser therapy may help. Antioxidant supplements are sometimes used to slow the progression of the disease.

Cornea disease occurs when the transparent part of the eye (cornea) becomes thick, flat and less smooth. Part of the eye may swell and cause cloudy vision, a result of cell degeneration on the inner surface of the cornea. To reduce the swelling and haziness, saline eye drops are sometimes used. In severe cases, corneal transplants may be necessary to restore vision.

Our eyes may become more sensitive to light, temperature and wind, causing excessive tearing. It is not a serious problem but can be uncomfortable. On the other hand, our eyes can become dry and irritated, especially in climates where the humidity is low. Most eye doctors recommend artificial tears. Living in the southwest, most of my friends and I use them as frequently as four times a day. Be careful to use only the products specified as eye lubricants.

I don't have to tell you how precious your sight is. That is why an annual or semi-annual eye examination is imperative for people in this age group. Early detection of an eye disease better enables your doctor to halt or retard its progress.

TASTE AND SMELL:

Loss of appetite is a common problem at this age. I am experiencing it now. Foods I once enjoyed no longer appeal to me. My capacity for food has diminished. I have gotten out of the habit of cooking each day. Sometimes, just the thought of turning on the oven and/or washing all those pots and pans, leads me to take the easy way out and eat a sandwich. After preparing meals for a family for so many years, I no longer have a desire to cook. However, I know how important good nutrition is at this stage of life. The time has come for me to take my own advice and make sure I get proper nutrition. Presently, my daily diet includes orange juice, cereal with milk and fruit and no-fat yogurt. Chicken, eggs (very little red meat), fresh fruit, and vegetables round out my daily food intake. Four to six small meals a day seems to work for me. I know I don't eat enough food to get all of the essential vitamins and minerals my body needs, so I take a daily multi-vitamin. Of course, it is best to get nutrients from the food you consume.

Sometimes, as we age, taste intensity diminishes. Some of us may be adding more salt to our food to make it taste better. Too much salt in your diet can be harmful, especially if you have high blood pressure. In addition, our sense of smell diminishes, making food less appealing. Try adding herbs and spices instead of salt.

Seniors are retaining their natural teeth longer than any previous generation. Some of you may not believe that maintaining good dental health at this stage of the game is important - think again. Not only is there a link between dental health and overall health, but dental problems can prevent you from chewing and digesting food efficiently. This can contribute to loss of appetite and in turn, weight loss. Diligent dental hygiene (see 61-75) doesn't take much time and effort, but the benefits are huge.

Previously, I have emphasized the importance of maintaining low body fat. However, at this age, being too thin can put you at risk. You need a little fat to draw from in case you become ill and cannot eat. Mal-nutrition among older adults is common. It is up to you to make an effort to get the nutrients your body requires.

YOUR MIND:

Good nutrition is essential to maintain a healthy brain. Eat plenty of fruits and vegetables, making sure you consume the daily-required vitamins and minerals. Vitamin E, an antioxidant, is especially important to help protect brain cells and blood vessels. Vitamin C, also an antioxidant, works to protect the capillaries. Because it is water soluble, it is not stored in the body for very long. It's best to consume it every day.

You need minerals, such as magnesium, copper, phosphorus and iron to maintain the nerve impulses in your brain, build hemoglobin and maintain metabolism. Despite the fact that our brains shrink by five to ten percent as we age, we still have about one hundred billion nerve cells (neurons) and billions of glial cells, which supply the neurons with nutrients. Neurotransmitters are the chemicals that transmit messages (electrical impulses) across junctions, called synopses. With age, this process slows down. Your instant recall may not be so instant anymore. That does not mean you are on your way to Dementia or Alzheimer's disease.

Exercise is essential to brain health. In addition to improved blood circulation, physical activity sharpens your senses and motor reflexes. Many senior centers offer both water and dry land classes either free of charge, or at a nominal fee. Seniors seem to love the mind-body exercises, such as Tai Chi or Ai Chi. (See EXERCISE). The social aspect of taking classes with other people your age, can be fun. If that doesn't appeal to you, simply walking several times a week will do the trick. Should you choose walking, I suggest that you start out slowly and work toward a faster pace and longer distance. First, walk the same distance a few times, and keep track of the time it takes. Make an effort to increase your pace each time you walk and when the faster pace becomes comfortable, increase the distance. You'll keep your juices flowing and increase your leg strength.

Don't think you are too old to do weight training. Dotty, my eighty-three year old friend, keeps a set of three-pound weights in her kitchen, so that she can work out when she is "waiting for the water to boil." In addition, she does all her own house and yard work and line dances for an hour and a half once a week. That is quite an aerobic workout!

Dotty keeps her mind active by writing. Presently, she is working on her memoirs for her grandchildren. While she was married to a career service man, they traveled the four corners of the earth. Her stories about her experiences in remote places are fascinating. What a great legacy to leave to her family!

Adequate sleep is every bit as important to your health and well-being as it ever was. It can mean the difference between feeling well and dragging yourself around just to get through the day. The amount of sleep you need is highly individual. Some need more than others do. How you feel is the best barometer to go by. Here are some suggestions to help you get the sleep you require:

- Go to bed at the same time every night.
- Avoid caffeine after 4 P.M.
- Avoid alcoholic beverages after 6 P.M.
- Avoid afternoon naps if they interfere with your night's sleep.
- Do something relaxing such as reading, listening to music or breathing exercises prior to bedtime.
- Try to clear your head of anything stressful.

Thanks to huge advances in medical science in the past few generations, we are living longer, healthier and more productive lives. Seniors now have an important role in society. Many of us are still in the work force. Politicians are hearing our concerns - since we became a large group to deal with. American culture is now beginning to recognize the value of wisdom and experience. Our media personalities are becoming more 'gray'. Youth worship is losing popularity. I can remember when you could not get a job if you were over forty. I also remember reading in a fashion magazine, that no woman over forty should wear pink or have long hair. Whoever wrote those things would cringe at today's seniors running around in jeans and sneakers.

Now that you have these bonus years, what are you going to do with them? My first thought is to take the best possible care of yourself. It would be ungrateful to the medical profession not to do so. Regular medical care, good nutrition, exercise and proper rest should be your top priorities. Your attitude toward your life can make or break your health and well-being.

A good example of a positive outlook on life, is my friend's ninety-three year old Aunt Bea. She worked full-time until she was eighty-five. She lives alone, exercises forty-five minutes each day, and sees to it that she eats five servings of fruits and vegetables a day. In short, she's taking the best possible care of herself. Her goal is to reach one hundred as both of her sisters did. They lived one hundred-three and one hundred-five years respectively. She is already planning her one hundredth birthday and looking forward to receiving a birthday card from the President of the United States, just as both her sisters did.

Eighty-seven year old Bernadette has the most unsinkable spirit I have ever seen in a human being. She has been battling cancer for four years and the surgery required to remove the cancer, left her with lymph edema in one of her legs. In order to keep the swelling down to a minimum, she must have it wrapped by a medical professional about twice a week. In addition, she goes alone by bus to Sloan Kettering Institute once a month for a check-up. Recently, she became afflicted with Shingles. Despite the pain and discomfort she endures from these conditions, she travels to Minnesota annually to visit her daughter, and on a regular basis, to Cape Cod, Massachusetts to visit her sister. Weather permitting, she walks in the park, three times a week, for about an hour. She's still the same person I have known and loved for many years. Everyone is drawn to her, including my children and grandchildren, because she's so much fun. That hasn't changed.

Jack LaLanne, a pioneer in the fitness business, showed up on my TV recently. Well into his nineties, he still wears his signature jumpsuit, showing off his trim and muscular physique. I still recall exercising along with him on TV every day back in the sixties and seventies. That was before I got into the fitness business myself. I thank him for keeping me fit during those years.

These *can* be golden years. It's up to you how you spend them. Watching my adult grandchildren graduate college, begin a career, get married and start families of their own, is a joy I never imagined. I don't know about you, but I plan to live each day to the fullest. I feel that it is my duty and responsibility to do so.

***

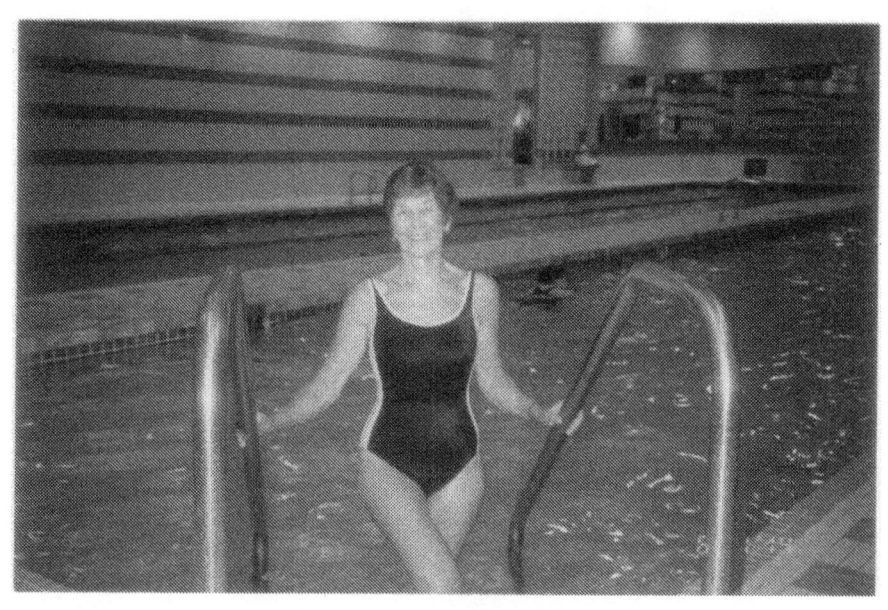

I hope you

have enjoyed your

journey with me

through a lifetime of fitness.

May you always be at

YOUR PERSONAL BEST.

Sincerely,

Marie McDonald

About the Book

When you get right down to it, most people do care about fitness – they are interested, but just haven't the first clue how to begin. Where and how do you learn just how to start, without appearing less than bright? All the new words we hear and read, no doubt having something to do with fitness, what do they mean? I mean really, Pilates, Ai Chi, Tai Chi – are they animal, vegetable or mineral. Help!

Help is here. The subtitle of this book is *A Common Sense Guide to Fitness for All Ages.* The book not only covers complete information on fitness training, but advice on weight control and diet, water exercises and abdominals and much more.

Also included is a complete section on attaining and maintaining fitness from birth through the Golden Years – all the way. People tend to give up, but they could improve their fitness, even with disabling conditions.

After you read the extremely enlightening and useful information in this book, you may very well call it Your Personal Fitness Handbook.